NARENDRA AND KUNDAN MEHTA

the face
lift massage

rejuvenate your skin and reduce fine lines and wrinkles

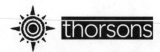
thorsons

Thorsons
An Imprint of HarperCollins*Publishers*
77–85 Fulham Palace Road
Hammersmith, London W6 8JB

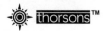

and Thorsons are trademarks of
HarperCollins*Publishers* Limited

The website address is:
www.thorsonselement.com

First published as *Indian Face Massage* by Element,
an imprint of HarperCollins*Publishers* 2001
This edition 2004

1 3 5 7 9 10 8 6 4 2

A catalogue record for this book is
available from the British Library

ISBN 0 00 715741 X

Photography by Guy Hearn
Illustrations by Jane Spencer
Medical illustration by Peter Cox Associates

Printed and bound in Great Britain by
Martins The Printers, Berwick upon Tweed

dedication

This book is dedicated with love to my Uncle Gopaldas and Auntie Bhanuben and their family for their continuous love and support.

acknowledgements

There are many people to whom we owe a great deal but as there are so many we have restricted ourselves here to those who have directly contributed to this book.

For researching and helping to write this book, Ranu Bhullar and Norman MacCallum.

Also other friends without whose help this wouldn't have been possible, Robert The, Lesley Hart, Charlotte Wayne. Belinda Budge, Nicky Vimpany and others at Thorsons. And finally our parents who have always been a constant source of encouragement throughout our careers.

authors' note

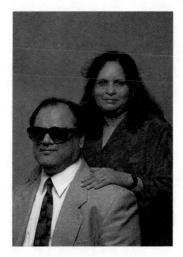

Not many people can maintain a happy marriage and work together but we share our love of life, knowledge, and each other to such an extent that work is always a great pleasure. As we have been working together and have studied various therapies we have taken a greater interest in face lift massage. We have taken our inspiration from both Eastern and Western forms of massage and adapted our own unique technique of face lift massage, which Kundan has been practicing for several years. We've now decided to share our knowledge with you by writing this book. It has been very challenging, as Kundan uses her intuition as part of her technique, which is hard to put into words, but we have done our best to do it justice.

In this book we have described a few simple and effective techniques to keep you looking and feeling younger for longer. The beauty of this therapy is that it is non-invasive and all you need is a willing partner with healing hands to follow the simple instructions. We believe everyone has healing hands and all you need to do is follow the instructions carefully and allow the healing to flow. A face lift massage is incredibly relaxing to receive and very easy to give. We've also shown that self-help facial exercises and changing your lifestyle can also greatly delay the signs of aging.

Kundan practices at the Eastern Health and Beauty Centre at the London Centre of Indian Champissage, 136 Holloway Road, London N7 8DD. Tel: 020 7609 3590, 020 7607 3331. Email: mehta@indianchampissage.com, www.indianchampissage.com. This is our second book. The first on *Indian Head Massage* is a great success and we hope this will be too.

contents

introduction

ancient wisdom, modern beauty

With the passing of time, your lifestyle and personal experiences, both good and
bad, can start to show on your face. From your early twenties onwards, every
laugh and frown that you express begins to leave its cruel imprint in the form of
tiny lines around your eyes and mouth. Add to this the effect of traffic pollution,
sunshine vacations, the stresses and strains of modern life, too many late nights,
and all the other abuses you've subjected your body to and, before you know it,
you're starting to look older than your years. The good news is – it doesn't have
to be like this.

We have devised a technique called face lift massage that can give you a natural
face-lift. With the simple moves shown in this book, you can delay the aging
process by means of facial massage, the stimulation of pressure points, natural
beauty treatments, and other well-proven techniques that have their origins in
ancient Indian traditions. This treatment not only helps to reverse many adverse
effects to your skin but can go a long way to delaying or preventing further
damage in the future. If that's not enough, a face lift massage can leave you
feeling relaxed, stress free, and at peace with the world. It sounds too good to be
true – but it does work!

Step by step, this book will help you get to know your skin, the underlying
tissues and the facial muscles, and show you what you can do to stay looking
younger for longer. Drawing on the wisdom of Ayurvedic healers, who practice
an Indian healthcare system dating back thousands of years, and combining this
with other tried and tested therapies, such as yoga, energy balancing, and
Ayurvedic massage, we will show you how to carry out a simple but effective
facial care program that will leave you looking and feeling rejuvenated,
energized, and ready for whatever life has in store.

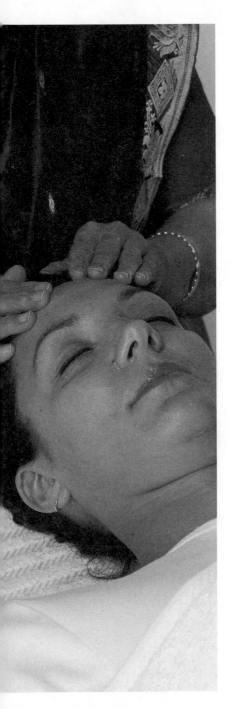

As well as our unique massage system and skincare routine, we offer practical advice on healthy eating, getting a good night's sleep, managing your stress levels, and regulating many other aspects of your lifestyle that can bring immediate – and lasting – benefits to your mind and body. Be warned – this book can change your life!

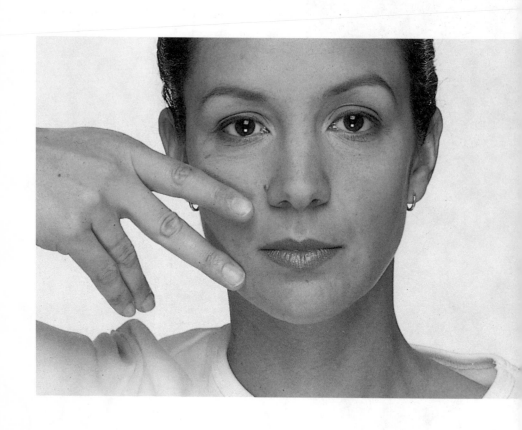

the art and science of face lift massage

what is facial rejuvenation?

Facial rejuvenation may sound like the stuff of science fiction but our system of beauty care draws on ancient wisdom and well-established techniques, combined with many modern approaches, to provide a truly "holistic" – or "whole body" – treatment.

This unique method requires no oils, equipment, surgery or drugs. All you need is a quiet, comfortable place to practice and a little time to spare. For some exercises, you'll need a pair of willing hands to massage you, or you can learn how to help others to look younger. Why not practice with a friend, partner or family member so you can all enjoy the benefits?

Under the hands of an expert, you can usually see a difference after just one treatment. But even a novice can make a dramatic improvement by helping to free up the restrictions in the tissues that are the principal underlying cause of lines, wrinkles, and sagging flesh. The more you practice, the sooner you'll see results, which in some cases can only be described as truly amazing. You'll clearly see how the skin has been rejuvenated – it looks "lifted up" and also feels softer and more supple.

how does it work?

In this modern, stress-filled world your mind can be busier than the rest of your body. This is often reflected in your face. Hectic thoughts and pent-up emotions cause the muscles of the face, neck, shoulders, and head to tighten and constrict. This can lead to chronic aches and pain, especially around the eyes, jaw, neck or shoulders, and is a warning sign that your body's natural energy is not flowing freely. Don't be confused by the term "natural energy." Many cultures believe that there are vital energy centers all over the body and that the flow of energy between these centers has a direct effect on a person's health and well-being. A blockage in the energy flow causes symptoms such as pain and fatigue and usually leads to disease. By using massage to release such blockages you'll find that not only has the discomfort gone but the energy now flows freely around your body, helping you to make better connections between your internal organ systems, thoughts, and emotions.

The seven chakra points

In India the body is said to contain seven main energy centers or chakras. If there is a blockage in any one of them it can cause an obstruction in the energy flow. This can build up and spiral to the head, leaving you feeling tense and imbalanced.

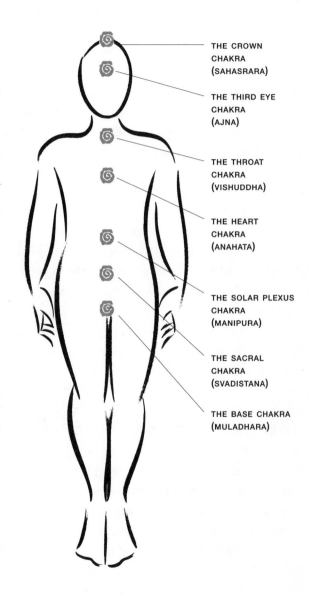

THE CROWN CHAKRA (SAHASRARA)

THE THIRD EYE CHAKRA (AJNA)

THE THROAT CHAKRA (VISHUDDHA)

THE HEART CHAKRA (ANAHATA)

THE SOLAR PLEXUS CHAKRA (MANIPURA)

THE SACRAL CHAKRA (SVADISTANA)

THE BASE CHAKRA (MULADHARA)

the magic of facial massage

For many Indian people, massage – including head massage and facial massage – is a daily part of their lives from the day they are born and is considered as important to health and beauty as diet and exercise. Facial massage is one of the most important elements of facial rejuvenation. It is like ironing with your fingers. Using repetitive finger movements along each wrinkle and also working on the underlying facial muscles, you can relieve tension in the muscles of the face, neck, and scalp, smoothing away lines and bringing elasticity and sheen back to the skin. You're left looking and feeling younger and happier as the stresses and strains of the day simply float away. You just can't help smiling after a facial massage because of the intense sense of contentment it induces.

Facial rejuvenation also works on the structure of the skin, to ease restrictions and lift up the face. Most of the skin is made up of connective tissue, which is formed from fibers of proteins such as collagen and elastin. These fibers weave together to form a flexible web-like structure. In younger tissues, the fibers slide past each other freely, giving suppleness and flexibility. But over time, toxic by-products build up in the skin, causing the fibers to lock together, so that the skin loses much of its mobility. Facial rejuvenation helps to release the tissues, gently allowing the connective tissue to regain its freedom and elasticity.

ancient theory – modern approach

The treatments we use in facial rejuvenation have mainly been drawn from ancient cultures but have been complemented by more modern methods. The main techniques we use come from Ayurveda. This ancient healing system has evolved over four thousand years and is one of the world's oldest forms of health care. The word Ayurveda is derived from two roots in Sanskrit: "vida," meaning "science" and "ayus," meaning "life," so it is usually translated as "the science of life." It is one of the first holistic therapies as it is concerned with the health of the individual at all levels – physical, emotional, and spiritual. It treats the patient and not the illness and aims both to prevent disease and promote good health.

Ayurveda informs us that individuals have their own distinctive balance of three types of subtle energies or doshas. These are vata dosha, pitta dosha, and kapha dosha. Although they regulate thousands of different functions in the mind-body system, they have three basic functions: vata controls movement, pitta controls metabolism (body chemistry), and kapha controls structure.

Ayurveda teaches that every cell in the body must contain all three energies. The body needs vata to breathe, for blood to circulate, for food to pass through the digestive tract, and for nerve impulses to travel to and from the brain. Pitta processes food, air, and water, and kapha holds the cells together to form muscle, fat, and bone. All these energies need to be in harmony to promote physical, emotional, and spiritual well-being. In individuals there is usually one particular dosha that is dominant in the constitution, and this influences the person's lifestyle. For example, Kapha types may need to eat certain foods, do particular exercises, and follow special routines in order to balance this dosha and so stay in good health.

Ayurveda places great emphasis on massage as being essential to health and beauty and people are advised to adopt it as a fundamental part of their daily routine. Just as we eat and sleep every day, so we should have a daily massage. Certain conditions can be treated by massage. For example, people who suffer from insomnia benefit from having a head and face massage, or massaging themselves, just before they go to bed. Massage also boosts the immune system by stimulating the production of white blood cells and antibodies. This strengthens bodily defence mechanisms and so increases resistance to viral and bacterial diseases. In India, babies are massaged from birth. The physical contact makes them feel nurtured and helps to ensure that they grow strong and healthy. Massage can work for you, too, helping you to look and feel revitalized, young, and beautiful.

beauty inside and out

Ayurveda shows us how to be beautiful inside and out and teaches that the two are related. Outer beauty is not just concerned with the way you look, but also includes posture, the way you move, and having a radiance that glows from within. Inner beauty relates to qualities such as your emotional state and mental abilities. The more you nurture yourself and learn to balance your inner and outer selves, the more insight you have on the world. Beauty evolves with age. As you get older, you learn to tap into a new source of beauty that comes from personal experience.

Ayurvedic facial massage gives amazing results. It relieves tension from areas that you had no idea were tense. After a massage you are left with a terrific feeling of well-being; your whole body feels totally relaxed and soothed. We owe a great deal to Ayurveda for the particular form of massage that we have developed. But we have also incorporated other therapies. Our system of facial massage includes other techniques that have now become separate modalities. These are yoga, polarity therapy, acupressure, and Swedish-style massage. Yoga, like Ayurveda, has its origins in ancient Hindu scriptures called the Vedas. It is a system for life that uses postures, special breathing methods, meditation, and other techniques to release and channel energy through the body. Polarity therapy stimulates and balances human energy fields – subtle patterns of electro-magnetic energy that surround the body. In polarity therapy, illness is viewed as a disturbance in these patterns and so health is restored by rebalancing the energy fields.

Reiki is a Japanese word meaning "universal life force energy". The "ki" part of the word is the same as "prana" in Hindi and "qi" or "chi" in Chinese and is the term used to describe the form of energy that underlies everything in the universe. Reiki is a system for channeling universal energy to others for the purpose of healing and is similar to the chakra energy balancing used in Ayurveda. Compared with many Eastern healing systems, Reiki is relatively new as it was only developed just over a hundred years ago.

Acupressure is closely related to acupuncture but instead of applying needles, practitioners use tapping, pressing, and rubbing actions to stimulate and rebalance energy pathways in the body.

Swedish-style massage involves more rigorous stroking and twisting actions of the hands to stimulate the skin, underlying tissues, and muscles. This form of massage works on specific areas to improve the condition of the skin, lift up the face, and relax the whole body. By combining all of these disciplines, we have developed a form of massage that is perfectly tailored to tackle the stresses and strains of our modern, fast-paced, Western lives.

benefits of face lift massage

Face lift massage proves that you don't need cosmetic surgery to look younger. You can work towards reversing the aging process by yourself, by getting a friend to help you, or by visiting a qualified therapist regularly – and there isn't a snip or tuck to be seen! Nor is there a need to use any of the expensive cosmetics that claim to offer the elixir of youth in a bottle. Wrinkles and expression lines are reduced to give you a more vibrant and youthful appearance. Your skin becomes softer, complexion and skin tone improve, bagginess, sagginess, and puffiness are reduced, and you'll notice the elasticity returning to your face.

These are the visible benefits. But you'll also notice that you feel more relaxed as tension is released from facial muscles and the adjacent tissues, leaving your face feeling more mobile and your mental attitude much more positive. Headaches and other tension-related symptoms often disappear. In addition, as your body's energy flow is improved, you are left with a sense of general well-being, confidence, and joy. Be prepared – you may well feel like hugging the people around you!

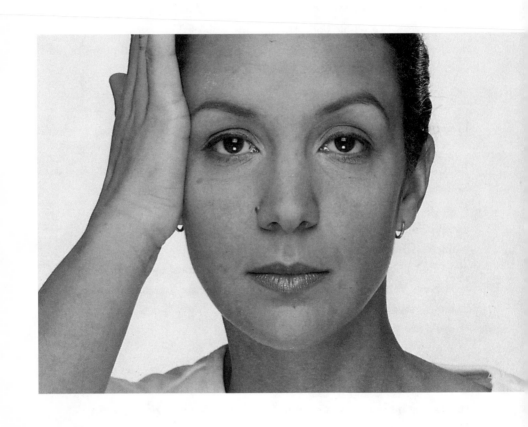

know your facial muscles

the force behind the face

The muscles of the face and neck vary in size and shape from the small, delicate structures around the upper lip to the large and powerful muscles of the neck and jaw.

All the muscles of the body are made up of long cords known as muscle fibers. These, in turn, are formed from smaller threads called myofibrils, which comprise even smaller strands, or filaments. The filaments slide past each other to contract the muscle and so exert a force. Your facial muscles play an important role in the way you look. They nestle closely together, sometimes even overlapping, and are joined to the skin in such a way that when they contract they pull the face into shape. By acting in combination they create the myriad expressions you use to reveal your conscious and unconscious feelings and interact with the world around you.

All muscles maintain a slight tension at all times to hold your position against the force of gravity. This is called muscle tone. However, when you're tense you tend to tighten the muscles for long periods, which impedes the flow of blood and starves them of oxygen and nutrients. For example, when driving a car in heavy traffic you tend to hunch over the wheel, developing tight, knotted muscles. Over time, the muscles become painfully tense and increasingly stiff. The best way to relax the muscles and restore their mobility is through massage and exercise. This is as true for the muscles of the face as it is for the rest of the body.

Facial muscles contract to reveal different expressions. If those expressions become habitual the muscles may stiffen up. Through massage you can release muscular tension and restore mobility to the face, so helping to restore your youthful features.

muscles of the face and neck

Before we go any further, you should get to know your face in more detail. It may help to find out about some of the muscles that lie underneath your skin and learn the names of a few of the major ones. The following are some of the most important muscles worked in facial massage.

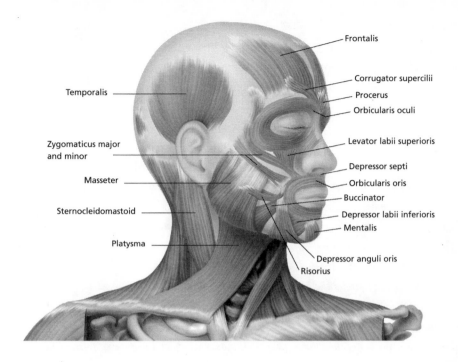

Frontalis

Corrugator supercilii

Procerus

Orbicularis oculi

Temporalis

Levator labii superioris

Depressor septi

Zygomaticus major
and minor

Orbicularis oris

Buccinator

Masseter

Depressor labii inferioris

Mentalis

Sternocleidomastoid

Platysma

Depressor anguli oris

Risorius

muscles of the face and neck

🌼 *Sternocleidomastoid – one of a pair of muscles on either side of the neck. It lifts your head when you're lying down, bends and tilts your head, and rotates your head sideways towards your shoulder.*

muscles around the eyes

🌼 *Corrugator supercilii – draws the eyebrows together in a frown and wrinkles the forehead vertically.*

🌼 *Frontalis – raises the eyebrows to show surprise and wrinkles the forehead skin horizontally.*

🌼 *Orbicularis oculi – narrows the eyes to frown and squint and closes the eyelid to wink. This muscle is the underlying cause of crow's feet.*

🌼 *Procerus – draws the eyebrows down and together.*

muscles of the nose

- ❀ *Depressor septi – depresses the nostrils.*
- ❀ *Levator labii superioris – flares the nostrils (and furrows the lips).*

muscles of the mouth

- ❀ *Buccinator – compresses the cheeks to blow a kiss, whistle, and suck.*
- ❀ *Depressor anguli oris – draws the corners of the mouth downwards and laterally to form a grimace.*
- ❀ *Depressor labii inferioris – draws the lower lip downwards to pout.*
- ❀ *Levator labii superioris – opens the lips, and raises and furrows the upper lip (and flares the nostrils).*
- ❀ *Mentalis – protrudes the lower lip and wrinkles the chin to express doubt.*
- ❀ *Orbicularis oris – closes the mouth and purses and protrudes the lips to kiss and whistle, and also pulls the lips against the teeth.*
- ❀ *Platysma – draws the corner of the mouth downwards and backwards to show horror.*
- ❀ *Risorius – draws the corner of the mouth outwards to grin.*
- ❀ *Zygomaticus major and minor – pulls the corner of the mouth upwards and outwards to smile.*

muscles of the jaw

- ❀ *Masseter – clenches the teeth and raises and closes the lower jaw tightly for chewing.*
- ❀ *Temporalis – raises the lower jaw and presses it against the upper jaw to aid chewing.*

get to know your face

The following exercises can help you to locate and identify some of the key muscles of the face.

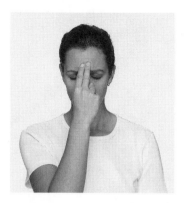

Place two fingers between your eyebrows and frown in a disapproving manner. You'll feel a combination of the Procerus, which lies just above the nose, and the Corrugator supercilii, located above the eyebrow.

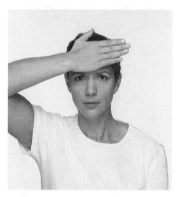

Place a hand flat against your forehead and scrunch up your forehead. You'll feel your hand being pulled up, mainly due to the contraction of the large Frontalis muscle. Working this muscle helps to increase oxygen and blood circulation through the forehead and around the eyes. This helps soften your brow, making you look more relaxed.

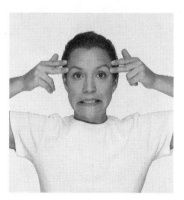

Place two fingers of both hands on either side of your head, slightly above and in front of your ears, and clench your teeth. You'll feel the wide Temporalis muscle, responsible for closing your jaw and aiding chewing.

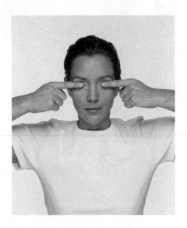

Close your eyes and gently place an index finger across the top of each eyelid. Keeping your eyes shut, widen your eyes as if trying to lift your eyelids. The delicate muscle you can feel is part of the Orbicularis Oculi, which encircles the eye.

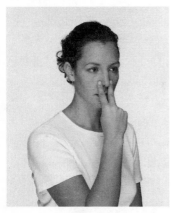

Separate the index and middle fingers of one hand to make a V shape. Place one finger on either side of your nose and try closing your nostrils. You'll feel the Compressor Naris.

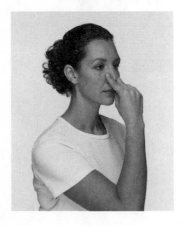

Now try flaring your nostrils. This involves the Depressor Septi and Levator Labii superioris.

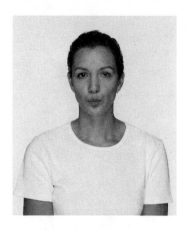

Purse your lips as if kissing and feel the circular muscle surrounding the mouth. This is the Orbicularis Oris.

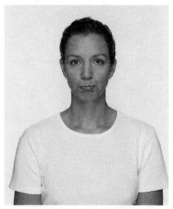

Protrude your lower lip and wrinkle your chin as if sulking. The muscle that controls this expression is the Mentalis.

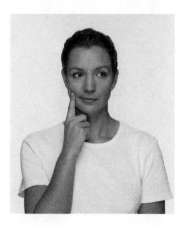

Place a finger slightly away from the corner of one side of your mouth and smile to that side. The muscles you can feel are the Zygomaticus major and minor.

express yourself

Now that you've become familiar with some of your facial muscles it's time to look at how they work together to create certain expressions. This is not just a learning process but also very good exercise. It's best to stand in front of a mirror so you can see how the muscles function. By doing these exercises regularly you'll become familiar with your face, your skin will take on a healthy glow, and there will be a fresh vitality about you. As soon as you can feel the muscles, let go and assume the next expression.

❁ *Begin by assuming the most neutral expression possible. Breathe slowly, relax your facial muscles, and clear your mind.*

❁ *Now imagine something fabulous has happened or that you've heard some great news. Let your face show the surprise. From this expression move on to the next one.*

❁ *Pretend you'd been desperately hoping something would happen but it hasn't. Let your face show your disappointment and sadness.*

❁ *Think of some of your happiest memories and show your happiness.*

❁ *We all get angry at times. Imagine someone has done something to make your blood boil. Let the mirror see how you feel.*

❁ *Now have a good laugh at yourself – pull faces or do whatever you need to do to make yourself laugh. Now we've come full circle so assume a neutral expression again.*

case study

Name: Rita

Age: 38

Occupation: Executive assistant

Rita first heard about the treatment from an article in a national newspaper and was interested because, quite naturally, she wanted to look as young as possible for as long as possible. As she believes prevention is better than cure, she started the therapy from a relatively young age to avoid wrinkles developing.

Rita was particularly concerned about the area around her eyes due to laughter lines and her tendency to pull the area when removing make-up. She was also worried about the lines on her forehead caused by her habitual expression.

After the first treatment Rita felt a sense of calm no other therapy had managed to achieve. She found the treatment very relaxing and felt great about being able to do something that she knew could keep her looking younger. Her face felt taut after each treatment but not in an uncomfortable way. After just one session her mother noticed something different about her but couldn't quite put her finger on it. After an initial course of eight treatments Rita felt she looked younger and her confidence grew because she was doing something to improve herself.

She definitely recommends face lift massage, as it's an excellent non-surgical way to look younger. Although she is 38 most people think she's about 30!

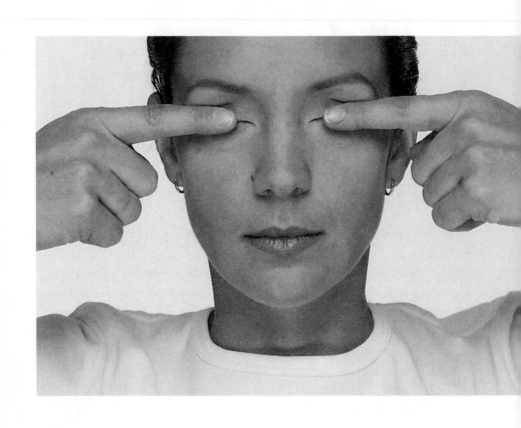

skin, lymph, and energy pathways

beauty is more than skin deep

Your face is made of many separate elements that fit together like a jigsaw to make up the face you see in the mirror. As you've already seen, the facial muscles play a vital part, and later on we will consider the role of the lymph system and also the energy pathways that, in all Eastern therapies, are considered crucial to your appearance and good health.

Nevertheless, the skin is also important and by learning how and why the skin changes with the passing years you'll start to appreciate why it is necessary to take good care of this vital organ. In the process, you'll discover new ways to delay, or reverse, the ravages of time and keep a youthful appearance for longer.

why skin is important

When you look at your reflection in the mirror usually the first thing you notice is the condition of your skin. You may have spent so long looking at your skin from a cosmetic point of view that you find it hard to think of the skin as a living organ. But the skin isn't there just to cover you up and make you look good. It has many vital functions that protect you and keep you alive. It is also a pretty accurate indicator of your state of health. When you feel dreadful, your skin usually looks off color. Healthy-looking skin is a sign of good physical health – and good mental health, too. Once you study the skin in detail, you'll begin to appreciate how complicated it is.

The skin is the body's largest organ. Spread out, it would cover about two square metres. It is constantly renewing itself, producing fresh cells and shedding dead ones as, for example, your clothes brush against your skin or you dry yourself with a towel. It is said that people shed what amounts to the entire surface of their skin once a week – no wonder that 80 percent of household dust is made up of human skin! If dead cells are allowed to accumulate they give the skin a dull, scaly appearance. So this is just one reason why a regular skin care regime, including exfoliation (see page 123), is important.

the role of the skin

The skin is highly intricate. Each tiny section of skin is packed with cells, nerves, blood vessels, hairs, sensory cells, and oil and sweat glands. The skin varies in thickness from only ⅕ in (0.5mm) around the eyes to ¼ in (6mm) or more on the soles of the feet, where it has to cope with the increased wear and tear of walking. It also thickens anywhere on the body where extra protection is needed, such as on the hands of manual workers. But the basic functions of the skin are the same wherever it is. These are: to regulate body temperature, protect against damage and disease, remove waste products, monitor your surroundings, and produce vitamin D.

temperature regulation

The skin plays a key role in regulating your temperature. If you get too hot, perhaps because you've just entered a warm environment or have been exercising hard, the blood vessels in the skin dilate to allow more blood to pass through them. This allows excess heat to escape from the surface of the body through convection and radiation. It is the increased flow of blood through the skin that makes you look flushed. As an extra measure against overheating, the sweat glands produce perspiration that seeps on to the surface of the skin through tiny pores. The perspiration absorbs heat as it evaporates and so helps to lower your temperature.

In cold weather, blood vessels in your skin contract to reduce the amount of blood flowing near the surface of your body and so conserve your heat. This is why some people look pale or almost blue when they're cold. In addition, the hairs on the skin stand up and this traps a layer of warm air around the body to provide extra insulation. When this happens, small bumps called goose pimples appear on the skin as tiny muscles pull the hairs upright.

protection

The skin covers virtually the entire body, providing a barrier that protects the underlying tissues from dehydration, friction, physical and chemical damage, and invasion by harmful organisms. The skin is relatively waterproof, although some moisture is absorbed when you take a bath – this causes the skin to swell, producing the wrinkling we notice after a long soak. The skin also contains sebaceous glands that produce an oily substance called sebum. This keeps the skin supple and lubricated and helps protect against moisture loss. The skin still loses some moisture, however, especially in the dry atmosphere of a modern centrally heated home or office, which is why you should apply moisturizer regularly to keep the skin supple. Sweat glands have an important defensive role, too. Sweat is slightly acidic and combines with sebum to produce a protective layer called the acid mantle that guards against bacteria and fungi. Sweat also contains an enzyme, lysozyme, that can destroy bacteria. In response to sunlight, some skin cells produce a dark-brown pigment, melanin, which blocks damaging ultraviolet radiation.

waste removal

Sweat glands not only help to control body temperature, they also excrete water, salts, and organic waste products in the sweat, so helping to regulate the body's salt and water levels and remove toxic substances. Regular exercise increases perspiration and so helps to flush out these toxins and prevent a harmful build-up.

environmental monitor

The skin is not only a barrier but also the main link between the body and the outside world, so its ability to monitor environmental conditions is of great importance. The skin houses nerve endings and receptors that detect stimuli related to temperature, touch, pressure, and damage. These nerve endings trigger impulses that travel to the central nervous system (CNS) to keep the brain informed about your surroundings, so you can make the appropriate response, such as pulling your hand away from a hot object. The connections between the skin and the nervous system are especially important during a massage. Even the lightest of touches is registered by the brain and has a direct and immediate influence on your state of mind and emotions; a pampering touch has a calming, soothing effect, while a firmer massage will leave you stimulated and invigorated.

production of vitamin d

Vitamin D is obtained from some foods, such as meat and fish, and is also formed in the body by the action of sunlight on the skin. This vitamin aids the absorption of calcium from the gut and so is needed for healthy teeth, bones, and nerves. Although you must protect the skin from the damaging effects of excessive ultraviolet radiation (see Chapter 8), regular moderate exposure to sunshine is vital to ensure an adequate intake of vitamin D.

skin structure

Bearing in mind just how important the skin is, it should come as no surprise to learn that this organ is not a shapeless mass of cells but has a complicated structure. The skin consists of two main layers; the outer one is the epidermis and the inner one is the dermis. The main function of the epidermis is to form a tough barrier against the outside world, while the dermis is a soft, thick cushion of connective tissue that lies directly below the epidermis and largely determines the way the skin looks. Both layers are constantly repairing and renewing themselves, but the dermis does so more slowly than the epidermis. Under the dermis is a layer of fat cells, known as adipose tissue or subcutaneous (below the skin) fat, which provides insulation and protective padding as well as a store of energy.

Just as the thickness of the skin varies slightly throughout the body, so does the structure. For example, you do not find hairs on the palms of the hands or the soles of the feet. Generally, though, the skin is pretty similar all over the body. If you examine the skin in more detail you can see what an amazing job it does.

The epidermis

The epidermis is sub-divided into four distinct layers:
the basal, spinous, granular, and cornified layers.

Basal layer: Cells here are attached to the basement membrane,
which separates the epidermis from the dermis. Basal cells
continually divide and grow to produce new cells that gradually
move up through the epidermal layers to the surface. The basal
layer also contains special cells, called melanocytes, that produce
the pigment melanin. Melanin not only acts as a sunscreen
against ultraviolet light but it also determines normal skin color,
being naturally more prevalent in darker-skinned people.

Spinous layer: Here, cells rising up from the basal layer
start to flatten out and produce a tough protein, keratin,
to protect the body from harm.

Granular layer: In this layer, the still-living cells
continue to flatten and fill with keratin but then
gradually lose their nuclei to become dead cells.

Cornified layer: This is the outermost layer of the epidermis
where the scale-like cells are made up almost entirely of
keratin. These cells are all dead and are constantly being
worn away and replaced by cells from below.

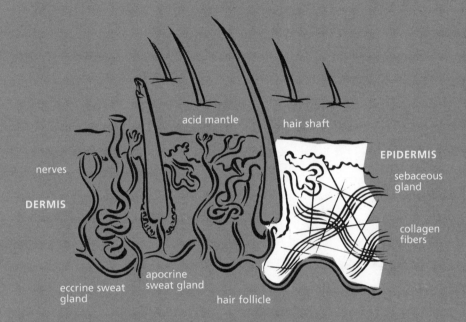

nerves

DERMIS

acid mantle

hair shaft

EPIDERMIS

sebaceous
gland

collagen
fibers

eccrine sweat
gland

apocrine
sweat gland

hair follicle

The dermis

The dermis is thicker than the epidermis. It consists mainly of connective tissue, which is made up of fibers of the proteins collagen and elastin and a non-fibrous gelatin-like material called ground substance or extracellular matrix (ECM) that fills spaces between the fibers. Moving through the matrix and among the fibers are fibroblast cells that manufacture the protein fibers and weave them together to form a web-like structure. These fibers often occur in bundles, made up of many fibrils lying parallel to one another, and they are very strong. They are found in all types of connective tissue such as bone, cartilage, tendon, and ligament.

The dermis contains blood vessels, which supply oxygen and nutrients to the skin and remove waste products, as well as special skin structures such as sensory receptors, nerve endings, sweat glands, and hair follicles – the deep pits that house the hairs. Each hair grows from the papilla, an area at the bottom of the follicle. Like skin, hair is made up mostly of keratin and is dead, except at its base, where new hair is constantly being formed. Each hair grows for about four years and then falls out and a new period of hair growth begins. Each follicle is surrounded by nerve endings that respond to the movement of the hair and can detect, for example, a light touch or a gentle breeze.

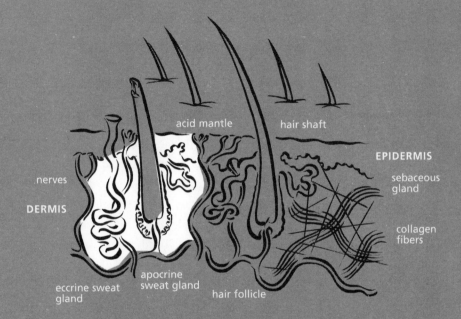

acid mantle

hair shaft

nerves

EPIDERMIS

DERMIS

sebaceous
gland

collagen
fibers

eccrine sweat
gland

apocrine
sweat gland

hair follicle

why does your skin age?

As we have already said, the dermis is mainly comprised of connective tissue so, to understand what happens to our skin as we get older, we need to look at this complex material in more detail. Connective tissue gives protection and support and is the most widely distributed material in the body. Under a microscope, the connective tissue of the dermis looks like a loose tangle of fibers. The main fibers are made up of the structural protein collagen and have great strength and suppleness. Collagen is the most abundant protein in the body and makes up about 70 percent of connective tissue. Collagen fibers are very tough and highly resistant to pulling forces although they do allow plenty of flexibility in the tissue.

Mixed up with the bundles of collagen fibers are thinner, more elastic fibers formed from a protein called elastin that increases the strength and flexibility of the connective tissue. Elastin fibers are smaller than collagen fibers and make up 5 percent of the dermis. They can be stretched by up to 150 percent of their relaxed length without breaking, which allows people to put on weight or expand during pregnancy without their skin tearing. Together, the two types of fibers give structure and suppleness to the skin, keeping the flesh smooth and taut.

Collagen and elastin bundles run in specific directions in different parts of the body. To discover the direction, pinch an area of skin and see which way it folds most easily into wrinkles. After a certain age, no pinching may be necessary as the wrinkles remain. A cut in the skin that separates parallel bundles of collagen fibers without damaging them heals with a fine line. But any injury that damages the fiber bundles forms a broad scar.

Although skin ages at a constant rate, the most noticeable effects occur from the late forties onwards. There are several reasons for this. When we are young the collagen and elastin fibers have tremendous strength and flexibility, but this gradually decreases. Over time, the fibroblast cells that produce collagen and elastin start to decline, so reducing the number of fibers present. Those fibers that are left may break apart while others can develop cross-links that bind them and lock them into place to form a shapeless matted tangle. This blocks the flow of fluid through the dermis, reducing its suppleness and preventing the fibers stretching and moving so freely with the muscles of the face.

Elastin fibers normally spring back into place when they've been stretched, which maintains skin tone. But with age they lose some of their elasticity, thicken into clumps, and become frayed. Once these fibers have hardened and shrunk, the skin tends to sag. Years of muscle action such as smiling and frowning can become imprinted on the skin as creases and wrinkles, especially on the forehead and around the eyes and mouth.

Another cause of skin aging on the face is a stiffening of the gelatin-like ground substance. The chains of protein molecules that make up this material get bound together, further reducing the skin's suppleness. As if that wasn't enough, the connective tissue of the dermis can glue the skin to the tissues surrounding the muscles and bones. This makes the face look drawn in, tight, and pinched. Other effects also occur over time. The layer of fat just below the surface of the skin gets thinner, underlying muscles start to shrink, and the water content of the skin declines, giving the rather loose and dry texture of aging skin. In addition, dead skin cells may not be replaced so uniformly when they are shed, giving an uneven appearance to the outer skin.

These age-related changes can't be prevented indefinitely. But there is much you can do to resist them. Facial exercises and massage (Chapters 4 & 5), coupled with a good skin care regime (Chapter 6), and sun protection (Chapter 8), help to keep the skin fibers supple for longer. A healthy diet (Chapter 7) ensures that the dermis gets all the nutrients it needs to build new fibers.

Underlying factors

Age-related changes to the skin are triggered by several factors
including excessive sun exposure; a build-up of harmful atoms called
free radicals; poor diet, such as excess sugar consumption; and, in
women in later life, a fall in the level of the hormone oestrogen.

Sun exposure: Ultraviolet rays penetrate deep into the skin,
drying the tissues and weakening the fibers, so accelerating
their disintegration.

Free radicals: These are unstable and highly destructive atoms. They
are a by-product of the normal chemical reactions in the cells that
release energy and are also produced by smoking, sunbathing, fried
foods, and industrial and traffic pollution. Although short-lived, free
radicals destabilize the molecules around them, causing damage to
living cells, especially in the skin, and leading to premature aging.

Excess sugar: This leads to sudden, steep rises in blood glucose levels
that can disrupt glucose regulation systems. The excess glucose binds
to proteins, in a process known as protein glycation, causing
irreversible structural changes to the skin, such as the cross-linking
of collagen fibers and other connective tissue damage associated
with aging. Protein glycation is a major problem for diabetics,
but also occurs in non-diabetics, underlining the importance
of a healthy diet.

Oestrogen: In women, the disintegration of the skin fibers is
accelerated in later life by a decline in oestrogen. Collagen in the
skin can fall by 30 percent during the first 10 years after menopause.

how massage can help

Facial massage is a valuable tool in resisting age-related changes. First of all, massage helps to relax the facial muscles. Muscular tension can restrict the blood vessels and obstruct the free flow of blood and other fluids to the tissues, so reducing the amount of nourishment the skin receives and preventing the removal of waste products. With massage, you can work the connective tissue to make space for the muscles to return to normal size, so releasing tension. After a few sessions you'll feel the tension ebbing away and notice a big difference in the condition of your skin.

Massage can also restore skin suppleness by helping to untangle collagen and elastin fibers, which then improves skin elasticity and helps to lift up the face. When you massage your face, or someone else's, feel with your fingers for signs that might indicate restricted tissue. This may seem difficult at first but, as with all things, practice makes perfect!

While muscles create the power to produce facial movements, connective tissue provides the structure and form to do so. For example, if you were to strip a body of its muscles, you would still be left with a clear shape of a human. But if you kept the muscles and stripped away the connective tissue, you would be left with a shapeless blob. When you look at diagrams of the muscles it's easy to see where they start and finish, but this isn't so straightforward with connective tissue.

Rather than beginning and ending at specific points, connective tissue is like a continuous sheath that surrounds the body. When massaging you have to develop the subtle skill of tracking the connective tissue. You'll find you have to untwist and rearrange it along several different planes at a time in order to release the tension. Because connective tissue forms a continuous network, when there is a restriction in one area, the impact of this can be felt in another area.

To understand this concept, imagine you're putting up a tent and securing it with pegs. If the pegs are spread evenly around the tent the canvas is smooth all over. But if you have more pegs on one side than another, the tension is uneven and one side becomes more taut. In much the same way, when massaging you are trying to ease restrictions in the connective tissue and even out the tension. The effect of this is often noticed elsewhere. For example, releasing a restriction in the neck can make the whole face look more relaxed.

the role of lymph

How many times have you looked at yourself in the morning and thought "why are my eyes so puffy and my skin so gray?" and "I must have slept very deeply because my pillow has left creases on my face." Well, some lines can be put down to your bed linen, but morning puffiness and lack of skin tone and color are partly due to the fact that your heart pumps blood more slowly at night, causing your circulation to slow down, but even more importantly, the flow of lymph drops dramatically while you sleep – and lymph plays a crucial part in the condition of the skin.

what is lymph?

Lymph is a clear, straw-colored fluid similar to plasma, the fluid part of blood. It starts out life as plasma, flowing through your arteries laden with oxygenated blood cells and nutrients to supply all your body's cells. Plasma leaks out of tiny blood vessels called capillaries and into spaces between the cells in the tissues to become tissue fluid. This bathes the cells, providing oxygen and nutrients essential for energy, growth, and renewal. It also removes wastes, bacteria, and toxins from the cells. The tissue fluid then drains into the lymphatic capillaries, where it becomes lymph.

Lymph flows in a closed network of vessels in a system that is completely separate from the blood circulation. The lymph capillaries join together to form lymph veins or lymphatics. The lymphatic system has no pump of its own, so to flow efficiently it relies on the movement of muscles, for example, when breathing or walking. As muscles contract they squeeze the lymph along the lymphatic vessels, which have valves to prevent the fluid flowing back. The lymph fluid eventually returns to the bloodstream via a connection between the lymphatic and venous systems, situated at the base of the neck.

You could think of lymph as a kind of internal irrigation system draining wastes from the tissues. At night, when this drainage system slows down, fluid builds up in the tissues. That's why your face can appear puffy first thing in the morning. Lack of physical exercise during the day also slows the flow of lymph. But that's not the only thing to watch out for – poor diet, pollution, and shallow breathing can all restrict lymphatic drainage.

One of the most important functions of lymph is its part in the body's defences. At intervals, the lymphatics empty into chambers called lymph nodes where the lymph is filtered and bacteria and other invading organisms are trapped and inactivated by white blood cells, or leukocytes, of the immune system. There are various kinds of leukocytes; some, such as the small lymphocytes, produce antibodies to destroy bacteria and viruses, while others are phagocytic cells that engulf and destroy foreign particles and organisms. Lymph must pass through at least two nodes before it is totally cleansed and can return to the bloodstream. If the lymph system gets overloaded you can see the effect in the condition of your skin, such as the appearance of spots, blackheads, and dry patches. While these problems can be treated easily, they needn't occur in the first place.

ancient wisdom

In Ayurveda, the lymphatic network is known as the kapha, or mucus-carrying, system. Thousands of years ago, Ayurvedic doctors developed a massage technique that included the manipulation of pressure points to balance the body's energy pathways. They thought that increasing kapha activity would improve the flow of nourishment to the bodily organs, aiding the movement of joints, and boosting patience, solidarity, stamina, and determination. When you look at the pressure points with a Western eye you'll notice that they correspond well with the position of the lymph nodes! How wise our ancestors were!

lymph and face lift massage

Face lift massage is a system that draws on much of the knowledge of the ancients. It involves massage and the application of pressure to certain points on the body to boost the drainage of lymph. Lymph can take time to thoroughly cleanse itself. In the meantime, the excess fluid under the skin and the build-up of toxins can be seen on the face, leaving it looking saggy, dull, gray, and puffy. Massaging the facial tissues helps to speed up lymph drainage and ensures that the vessels are cleansed of waste products that have not been removed naturally. There are important lymph nodes in the armpits, groin, and the back of the knees, but many nodes are in the neck, and by unblocking these you'll soon see a difference in your face.

Many of the lymph vessels are close to the surface of the skin, so you'll find that just a little effort has a major impact. In the long term, you'll notice your complexion is starting to glow and you'll have a more resilient immune system. Massage is a sure-fire way of getting the blood system moving efficiently, too. You'll quickly notice the color returning to your face as an indication that blood is now flowing more freely.

self help

You can give yourself a short massage to help lymphatic drainage and improve the condition of the skin on your face while also leaving you feeling relaxed. If you do these exercises regularly you'll soon notice a difference in your complexion. You may find that certain areas in your neck feel a little swollen, but this is normal as it means that toxins have been moved to the lymph nodes where they can be eliminated.

To help your hands slide, you may wish to rub a little oil into the palms of your hands. You could try a base oil such as almond or sesame oil, which you can find in most natural remedy shops, or just a few drops of olive oil may suit your skin. Avoid nut-based oils if you're allergic to nuts, as oil is absorbed by the skin. If you have overly greasy skin or acne it may be better not to use any additional oils.

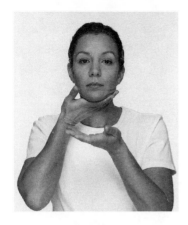

Using both hands alternately, sweep your neck upwards to the jawbone. Do this all around your neck, starting at one side and gradually moving along to the other.

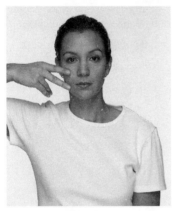

Separate the index and middle fingers of one hand to form a V shape. Place your index finger horizontally above your lips and your middle finger below your lips, just above the chin. Applying light pressure, slide your fingers out towards your ear. Repeat this with the other hand.

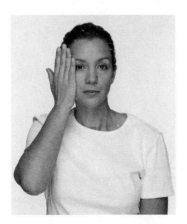

Place your fingers together. Pointing upwards, use the edge of your little fingers to apply pressure to the area next to your nose and mouth. Gently releasing the pressure, roll your hands across your face and slide your hands towards your ears. Hold the pressure for a few seconds.

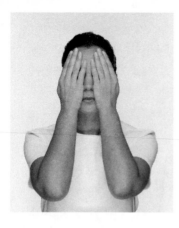

Close your eyes and place the whole of both hands over your face. Apply firm pressure to your face, hold for a few seconds.

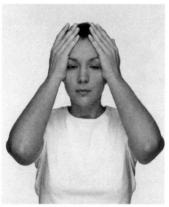

Now move your hands along and repeat, making sure you cover the whole of your face from neck to hairline.

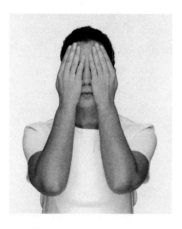

Finish by cupping your hands over your face and resting for a minute.

energy balancing

Another ancient tradition, acupuncture, also works on the lymphatic system. When you look at a map of acupuncture points, they correspond quite well to the position of the lymph nodes. It is interesting that both traditions of Ayurveda and acupuncture have located healing points that correspond to lymph nodes. Part of the philosophy behind acupuncture is that disorders arise because of an imbalance in the body's energy fields. You can rebalance these fields by manipulating the intercellular tissue fluid and lymph with needles, heat or massage. Both Ayurveda and acupuncture practitioners believe that lymph plays an important part in rebalancing the body's energy pathways – although they have their own methods for achieving this – and both believe that the role of health care should be preventative. Western doctors tend to concentrate on the chemical constituents of lymph, but it might be useful for them to study its effects on the body's energy pathways as well.

Acupressure works in a broadly similar way to acupuncture, but involves simple hand pressure rather than the use of needles. The results may not be as rapid as acupuncture, but the treatment is non-invasive and if practiced on a regular basis, can be even more effective.

Acupressure stems from a whole-body system of healing that has been practiced in China for over four thousand years. This system has been so successful it has spread throughout Asia and is now widely used in Korea, Japan, and Vietnam, as well as its mother country. Many Oriental women today use acupressure to stay looking young. To discover its rejuvenating power, you need to understand the principles of "yin and yang" and the vital energy "qi."

yin and yang

There have been many meanings given to the terms "yin" and "yang" but the most poetic arise from their literal translation: yin means "the shady side of the hill" and yang means "the sunny side of the hill." Yin relates to those aspects of matter that are dark, cool, heavy, and still, and yang relates to those that are hot, light, moving, and on fire. One cannot exist without the other and both form part of the same thing.

According to Chinese philosophy, everything around us is based upon yin being dominant at certain times and yang at others. As one grows stronger the other weakens. For example, yin dominates in winter but begins to weaken towards spring as yang reaches its peak in summer. As winter approaches, yin becomes dominant again. There is a similar "see-saw" effect in the body: if there is an increase in heat, or yang, it causes the fluids, or yin, to dry out.

Traditional Chinese medicine (TCM) believes that an imbalance between yin and yang leads to disharmony and disease. These ideas are similar to those of Ayurveda, which believes that health is maintained by keeping the doshas in balance. To achieve a balance between yin and yang, TCM seeks to improve the movement of body fluids such as blood and lymph and to stimulate the flow of "qi" energy.

qi or vital energy

Qi (pronounced chi) is the equivalent of prana in Hindi. According to ancient yogic beliefs, prana is the life force or vital energy that is inherent in everything. It is a subtle form of energy that is carried in air, food, water, and sunlight and animates all forms of matter. Prana is the life force that connects mind, body, and spirit. The ancient Chinese recognized a similar concept which they named "qi." They believed that everything, both living and non-living, is surrounded by qi. As qi flows through you, it forms a continuous matrix that links and feeds you with energy and determines the quality of your life processes from conception to death.

A smooth and uninterrupted flow of qi energy through your body is vital for health. When you look at a healthy person you can see the effect of qi by the "shine" on their skin. But if someone has a low level of qi, sickness and disease will result. Death is said to be marked by a total absence of qi. There is a special relationship between qi and body fluids such as lymph and blood. The circulating fluids nourish qi and influence its yin/yang balance and at the same time qi "energizes" the fluids.

the meridians

The vital energies of heaven and earth communicate with and flow along clearly defined, orderly, interconnected pathways in the body called "jing-luo," which translates as "meridians." The meridians carry qi. They are energy pathways forming an invisible network that links every part of your body. There are 12 principal meridians, each connected with, and giving energy to, a particular organ or system in the body.

Qi flows both "externally," meaning it circulates along meridians that are situated close to the surface of the body but below the skin, and also "internally," dispersing into broad webs of energy within the deeper tissues and organs. It nourishes every cell, nerve, muscle, bone, tissue, organ, and system with the energy vital for the proper maintenance and functioning of each part of the human body.

The meridians integrate and regulate the energy functions of the systems of the body by adjusting the deficiencies and excesses of qi. As qi flows through the body, each organ uses what it needs to function and then adds to the general flow of energy. If the flow of qi throughout the 12 meridians is smooth and unblocked and each one receives a balanced level of qi, then the body works well. But if the qi flow stops or is impaired in any way this results in pain, emotional, mental or physical distress, and disease. Acupressure is one of the ways used to treat blockages of qi. Massaging specific acupressure points on the meridians frees the flow of qi in the body as well as improving its quantity and quality.

practical approach

So that's the theory – now the practice. Facial acupressure involves stimulating certain points by pressing down with the tip of your thumb or your finger. By doing this you'll encourage qi to flow more freely. There are two techniques you could try. One involves stroking the face with very light pressure from the fingertips and the other uses the thumb tip or fingertip as a pump on the skin for about two minutes. Alternatively you could rotate the tip in small, circular movements to release blocked energy flows and relieve local muscular tension.

You can try an acupressure routine at home on yourself. All you need to do is study the picture opposite. Keep it in front of you for your first few treatments and then you should know your face well enough to continue without it. Remove any make-up and your contact lenses, if you wear them. Shut off all communication with the outside world and sit in front of a mirror in a very quiet place. Begin by rubbing your hands together to warm them. Work on the main acupressure points, moving from the hairline down to the neck. The points feel like small indentations under the skin. Practice this at least once a day, preferably in the morning, on rising.

As you become more familiar with the technique, you may notice that the skin at these points feels softer than the surrounding areas. Press down with a light pressure and then rotate your finger in little circles, taking care not to stretch or pull the skin. If you want even lighter pressure use your middle finger, as this is not as strong as your index finger. Hold down for five seconds. If this feels uncomfortable it might be a sign that there is a blockage along one of the meridians. If you continue to do this regularly the blockage should clear with time. However, if you feel any pain you should stop. Concentrate on the areas you are most concerned about. For example, if you have wrinkles around your eyes or lines across your forehead treat the relevant acupressure point three times.

1 Governor Vessel

2 Governor Vessel

3 Stomach

4 Gall Bladder

5 Forehead (Extra)

6 Urinary Bladder

7 Eyebrow (Extra)

8 Triple Heater

9 Gall Bladder

10 Stomach

11 Triple Heater

12 Small Intestine

13 Gall Bladder

14 Stomach

15 Large Intestine

16 Governor Vessel

17 Stomach

18 Stomach

19 Conception Vessel

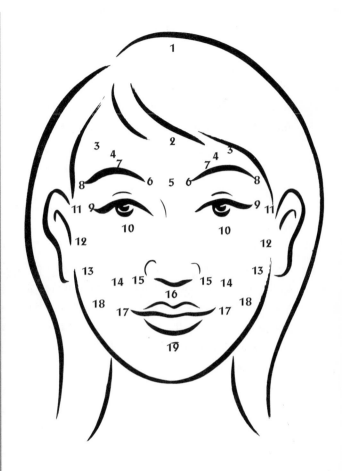

There are four different techniques for stimulating acupressure points. You can use any combination of the four that feels right for you:

- ✿ *Press down for a few seconds with a fingertip.*
- ✿ *Stroke your face with very light pressure from your fingertips.*
- ✿ *Use your thumb tip or fingertip as a pump on the skin for about two minutes.*
- ✿ *Rotate your fingertip in small circular movements.*

Acupressure is of most benefit when performed regularly. If you're treating yourself, or someone is treating you, remember to relax and breathe slowly. If you're treating yourself you should stop from time to time to check that you're not straining your arm.

Don't be too worried about finding the exact point since the body is an inter-related energy system and applying pressure anywhere on the skin surface will not only stimulate the local nerves and tissues but will also transmit a subtle energy throughout all 12 meridians – just like throwing a stone into a pool. With practice and intuition you'll discover that these points become easier to find. In fact, your fingers may seem to know where to go by themselves as they become sensitive to the energy flow.

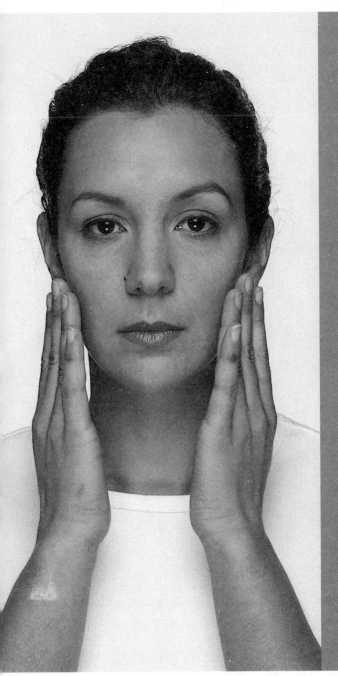

Warning

**Do not massage
someone who has
cancer or any serious
illness including an
active infection as
this can spread the
malignant cells and
micro-organisms
around the body
and interfere
with the body's
immune system.**

ⓑ

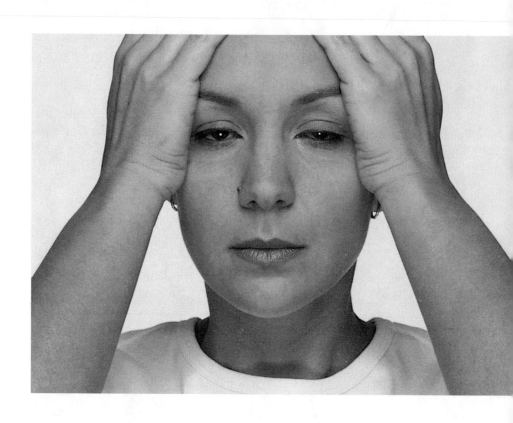

personal face exercises

holding back the clock

You have dozens of muscles in your face and, just like other muscles in your body, it is important to use them actively every day to strengthen them and keep them supple and toned. As we explained in Chapter 2, one way to exercise your facial muscles is to stand in front of a mirror and practice different kinds of expressions – laughing, smiling, frowning, and surprise – so all the muscles used in these actions get a good workout.

But there are specific exercises you can also do to tone individual muscles and the connective tissue.

As most people lead busy lives, we're not suggesting you find the time to do all the exercises. Just choose as many as you can realistically fit in to a normal day, concentrating on the areas you're most concerned about, and make it a daily routine. Perhaps you're particularly sensitive about one area of the face but not so worried about others. Whatever the case may be, we are now going to arm you with the techniques you need to deal with these issues. These exercises are not only designed to tackle problem areas that have already developed, but are useful preventative measures. In addition, they help to relieve stress, anxiety, and tension.

Many of these exercises can take a little time to get used to, and you may find that some muscles need more work than others, so you might not get immediate results. But facial muscles are very responsive and you'll soon notice an improvement. The earlier you start, the sooner the results will show. As with any exercise program, it's important to keep to a regular routine and persevere, even when you don't feel in the mood. Only then will you see a difference. Take care to do the exercises correctly or you may create more problems than you solve. Once you start to see a change you'll wonder why everyone who wants to stay young-looking doesn't take a few minutes out each day for a facial keep-fit session.

Your complexion – and what it may mean

Ayurvedic healers believe that the face acts like a window revealing the health of the body. Before you work on your face, study your reflection in the mirror and look for signs that could indicate deep-seated problems, such as a build-up of toxins. The following tips may help you to interpret the signs. If anything you notice causes concern, consult your physician or therapist.

Bags under the eyes: This may mean you are not getting enough sleep. If so, see pages 165–8 for advice. It might also indicate that the organs responsible for waste removal, particularly the kidneys, are overworked. Cut down on tea, coffee, and alcohol and drink lots of water, herbal teas, and fruit juice.

Deep lines on either side of the mouth: Is a long-running personal issue making you feel resentful? This can contort your face into a permanent pout. If so, deal with it and don't let it drag on. Chronic indigestion can also cause a hangdog expression.

Flushed: Have your blood pressure and heart rate checked. Flushes are common in women in later life because of hormonal changes.

Gray or dull skin: This may indicate a build-up of toxins in the body, perhaps due to excess smoking or drinking, which both create dehydration. Cut down or give up.

Oily skin: Your diet may contain too much fat – especially saturated fat – and processed food (see page 149). Cut down on fatty foods and increase your intake of high-fiber carbohydrates, fruit, and vegetables.

Pimples: This might indicate an allergy or there may be a build-up of toxins in your blood that your body is trying to eliminate. Consider a change of diet and eat more fiber, fruit, and vegetables.

White or unusually pale: If you're also feeling tired, this may be because your diet is lacking iron, leading to iron-deficiency anaemia. Increase your consumption of iron-rich foods, such as dried fruit, green leafy vegetables, liver, oily fish, pulses, shellfish, and tofu. Vitamin C aids absorption of iron, so include in your meals plenty of foods that are rich in this nutrient (see page 142).

warming up

Before beginning an exercise program always warm up first. Have a brisk walk, or jog, or run on the spot for five minutes; your skin and muscles are more supple when they're warm. Put on loose clothing, make sure the room is warm, and find a firm, comfortable seat.

Hold each move for up to five seconds and repeat up to five times.

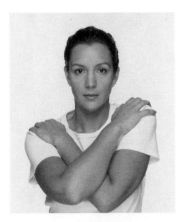

Start by loosening your shoulders. Place a hand on each shoulder and move your elbows clockwise, first one at a time and then both together.

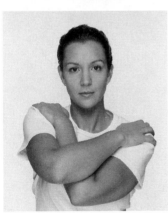

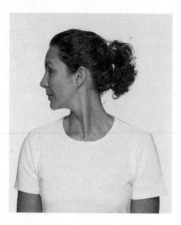

With your head vertical, turn to look over your left shoulder and then the right.

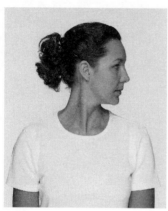

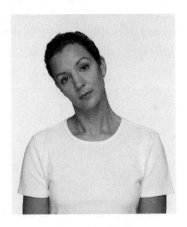

Looking straight ahead, slowly tilt your head from one side to the other, until you feel more flexible.

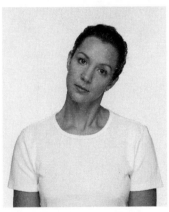

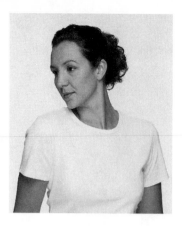

With your hands by your sides, swing your shoulders to meet your chin, first to the left and then to the right.

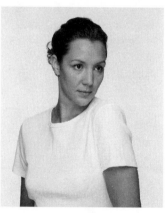

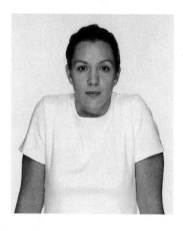

Raise your shoulders to your ears and then let them drop. Finish the warm-up by shaking out.

relaxing

Most of us store tension in our faces – in this stress-filled world of ours it's hard not to. But if left unresolved this tension can block the free flow of blood and lymph through the facial tissues and muscles leading to puffy, sagging skin and wrinkles. To help you relax your face try these steps.

Hold each move for up to five seconds and repeat up to five times.

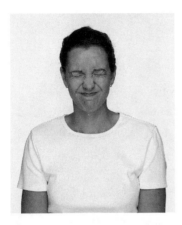

Scrunch up your face as tightly as you can and then relax and let it go back to normal.

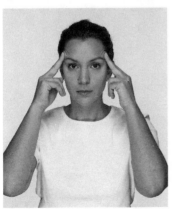

Place your hands on either side of your head and, with your fingers, do small circular movements to work the Temporalis muscles (on the sides of the head, just in front of the temples).

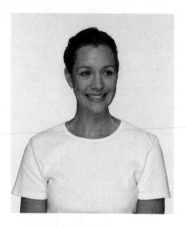

Let your jaw drop and, while breathing slowly, make the biggest smile you can and hold it for as long as possible. This is particularly satisfying as it releases a lot of deep-seated tension.

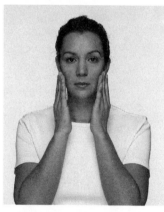

Search your face with your fingertips for any remaining pockets of tension you may have missed so you can release them by using light, circular movements.

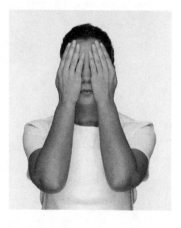

To finish, gently rest both hands on your face to give yourself warm energy.

tackling problem areas

Now you are ready to deal with specific areas of your face that may be giving you cause for concern.

forehead

If you have a tendency to frown, it's surprising how quickly permanent lines can begin to appear on your forehead. But there's no need to worry – you can do something about it.

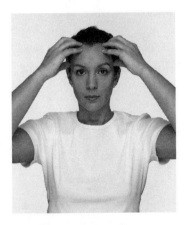

Place your fingers on your scalp and make small circular movements. This releases a lot of tension in the scalp – a major cause of worry lines.

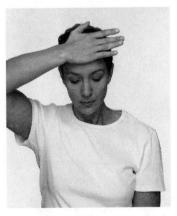

Press your hand against the top of your hairline to provide slight resistance and tilt your forehead slightly to look down. You should feel the skin of the forehead stretching. Now relax. This helps to reduce wrinkles and tone the skin.

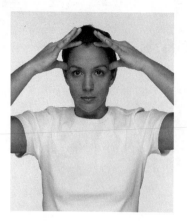

Place your thumbs on your temples and your index fingers at the top of your hairline. Push your index fingers up and your thumbs outwards to give yourself a stretched look. If you gather any skin you are doing it incorrectly.

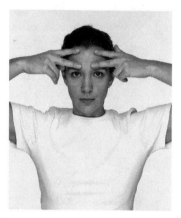

Place the fingertips of both hands above and below a line across the forehead. Gently pull the skin tight over the line.

The eyes are in use all day long, and as the windows to the soul they can often show signs of tension. If left unchecked, the area around the eyes begins to show the first signs of aging. Yoga has some simple exercises that can keep the eye area toned and relaxed.

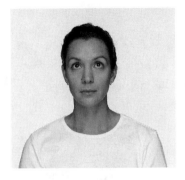

Trying not to move your head from the vertical, look up then down.

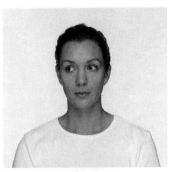

Look out of the corner of your eyes, first to the right, then to the left.

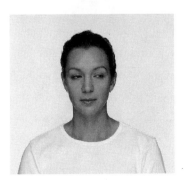

Congested lymph around the eyes can create new lines and deepen existing ones. If you've already noticed the march of time in the form of crow's feet and bags under the eyes, try the following exercises. They can help reduce these problems by easing the congestion. The skin around this region is very delicate, so be even gentler than you were with the rest of your face.

Hold each move for up to five seconds and repeat up to five times.

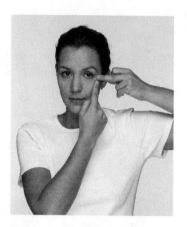

Place the index finger of one hand and the middle finger of the other on either side of a crow's foot wrinkle (corner of the eye) and press gently.

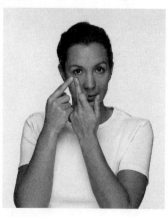

Place the index finger of one hand and the middle finger of the other on either side of a bag under one eye. Press down carefully and gently. Repeat with the other eye.

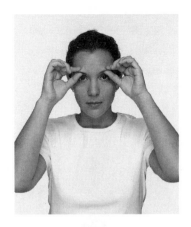

Grasp the skin on either side of
the eyebrow and roll it between your fingertips.
This releases the tension that can cause crow's feet.

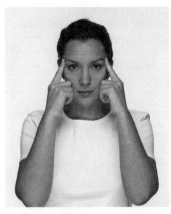

Place your index fingers on the ends of your
eyebrows above the outer corners of the eyes.
Gently stretch upwards and hold. Then release.
This can help to reduce crow's feet.

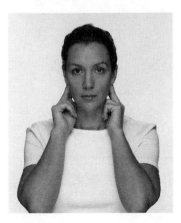

You wouldn't expect the area behind your ears to
have any connection with your eyes, but it does. By
massaging this area you help to remove any
lymphatic congestion that may have built up and
can cause bags to develop under the eyes. Place
your fingertips on the area behind your ears and
massage with gentle circular movements.

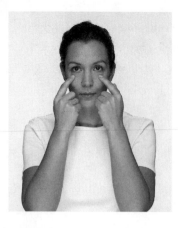

Use the index finger of each hand to make small circular movements, working from a corner of the eye around the eye socket and back to the corner of the eye.

Gravity is no friend of the eyes. Over time it can cause low eyebrows or drooping eyelids. As the eyes are such an important focal point of the face, this can have a dramatic aging effect. You can help prevent this by exercising the eyebrows and upper eyelids.

Repeat these moves up to five times.

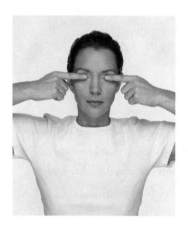

Close your eyes and place your index fingers across your eyelids. Applying gentle resistance to your eyelids with your fingers, try to open your eyes. This strengthens and tones the delicate eyelid muscles.

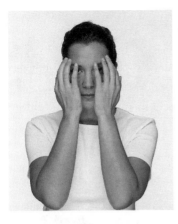

With your fingertips, tap backwards and forwards along the eyebrow. This releases tension.

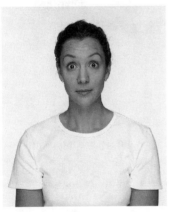

Raise your eyebrows as high as you can. Open your eyes as wide as you can. Slowly lower your eyebrows and relax.

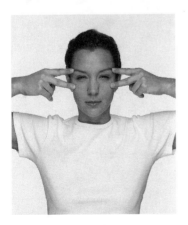

Create a V shape with the index and middle finger of each hand and place the fingers on either side of each eye. Try to squint using the fingers as resistance. This builds up the muscles in the area.

mouth

Your mouth works hard in enabling you to communicate, chew food, and show your mood. As the years go by, the smiling muscles on either side of the mouth can lose their tone, making the corners of the mouth turn down and look as though you're constantly sulking. Toning these muscles can help to level out the mouth.

Hold each move for up to five seconds and repeat up to five times, unless instructed otherwise.

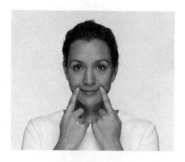

Place your index fingers on the corners of your mouth and tense the corners into an upward smile, using the fingers as gentle resistance. Now relax.

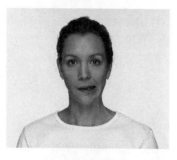

With your mouth open slightly, bring the corner of the left side of the mouth out as far as possible. Now do this with the right side of your mouth.

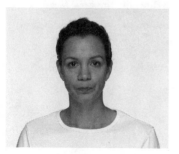

Puff up both cheeks and hold for up to five seconds. Release slowly. This helps to reduce laughter lines.

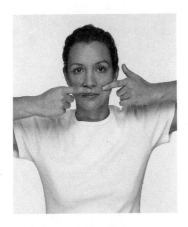

Using the index fingers of both hands, place one finger above the middle of your lip and the other above the laughter lines on one side of your mouth and gently stretch the skin upwards. Do this on the other side. Don't place your finger on the laughter lines as this can make the problem worse.

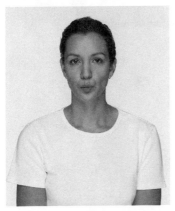

Pucker up your lips as far as they will go and make 10 "air kisses." This is another good exercise for laughter lines and can enhance your mood, as well as your appearance.

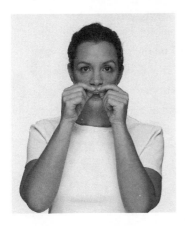

Place your thumbs under your top lip with the thumbnails resting against your gums. Feeling very relaxed, gently pull your upper lip down over your thumbs. Hold and gently release. Gradually repeat this along the length of your lip. This helps to erase the lines on the upper lip.

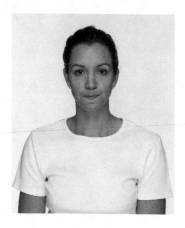

With your mouth closed, inflate your upper lip and hold.

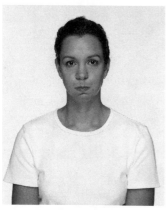

Now inflate the lower lip and hold.

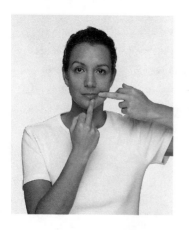

Smile to stretch your lips. Press the middle finger of your right hand on the right-hand corner of your mouth. Using the middle finger of your left hand, make small circular movements right along the edge of the bottom lip. Swap hands to work on the left-hand side of the mouth.

double chin and jowls

That old mischief-maker gravity can cause the muscles underneath the chin to lose tone and start to sag, giving the appearance of a double chin. These exercises can help to tone the area.

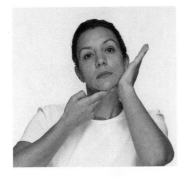

Using the index and middle finger of one hand, gently hold the skin of your jowl. With the other hand, using the ball at the base of the thumb, gently twist your wrist in an upward movement. Begin in the middle of the chin and work up the jaw line. Move along the jaw line and repeat on one side of the face three times. Then work the other side. This helps to reduce bagginess on the jaw line.

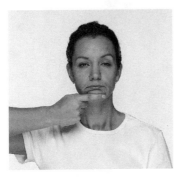

Place your index finger horizontally across your chin and, using it as gentle resistance, push upwards until you feel your jaw muscles tighten.

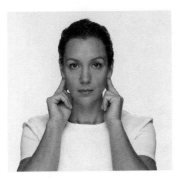

Place your index and middle fingers behind your earlobe and massage in a circular movement downwards. This encourages lymph drainage and helps to reduce sagginess around the jowls.

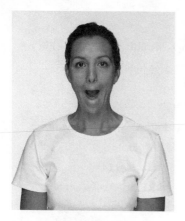

Open your mouth and pull your lower lip over your bottom teeth. Now open and close your mouth as if trying to scoop something up with your jaw. You really need to work the jaw hard to tone the muscles.

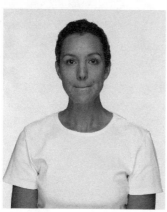

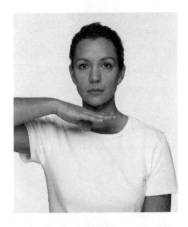

Use the back of your hand to tap or gently slap under your chin. Repeat with the other hand and increase the speed.

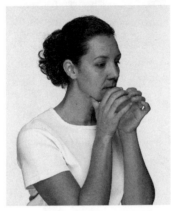

Place both thumbs under your chin to provide gentle resistance and push your chin down. Continue this symmetrically around the jaw line. This will tone up the chin muscles and help reduce a double chin.

neck

The skin of the neck is very thin and can slowly lose its natural elasticity and smoothness, drying out and becoming crêpe-like over time. In addition, lines can appear, slowly deepening the creases. The following exercises can help to remedy the problem.

Unless otherwise instructed, repeat each exercise up to five times, holding each one for up to five seconds.

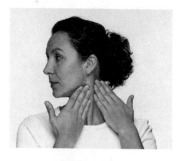

Turn your head to one side. Using both hands, hold the flesh on either side of the sternocleido-mastoid (the long horizontal muscle on the side of the neck, just under the jaw) until you feel a gentle throbbing (this is known as the healing pulse. See page 95). Continue up the muscle. Turn your head to the other side and repeat on that side.

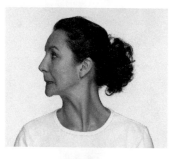

Keeping your neck muscles tense, slowly turn your head from side to side.

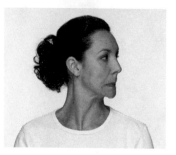

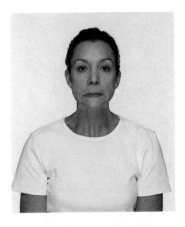

Keeping your head straight, tense your neck muscles and stick your neck out slowly, then bring it right back.

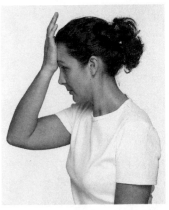

Place one hand on your forehead and push your head forwards using your hand as gentle resistance.

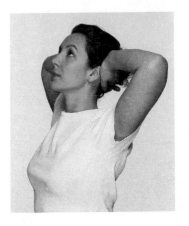

Now put your hands on the back of your head and push backwards.

nose

Believe it or not, your nose continues to grow as you get older. The tip drops and widens with age. The following exercises help to shorten and narrow the tip. If you feel particularly conscious about your nose, repeat the first two exercises more than once a day.

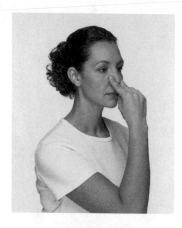

Gently hold your nostrils between your index and middle finger to offer gentle resistance and flare your nostrils as you slowly breathe in. Now slowly breathe out.

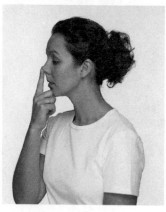

This exercise works on the Depressor septii muscle. Using your index finger, push the tip of your nose up and hold it firmly in place. Now pull your upper lip down over your teeth and hold for a second before releasing.

general complexion

If you have greasy or combination skin you may notice that there are open pores around your nose. The following exercise not only helps to reduce them, it also clears nasal congestion and aids lymphatic drainage.

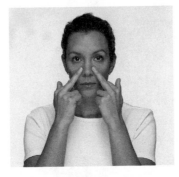

Using the middle fingers of both hands, make small circular movements from the top of the bridge of the nose down towards the nostrils. You may actually feel the lymph draining under your fingertips.

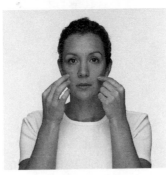

Use the thumbs and index fingers of both hands to gently pluck and pinch all over your face. This helps to improve the circulation and the general condition of your skin.

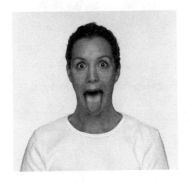

Sit up straight and look directly ahead. Open your eyes as wide as you can and stick your tongue out and down as far as it will go towards your chin. Hold this position for as long as you feel comfortable. Release and relax. Repeat five times.

five-step face lift

You may prefer an all-over facial work-out that won't take up too much time. If so, the following routine is specifically designed for people like you. Do this before applying your makeup in the morning, or after cleansing before bedtime.

Depending on your mood and the time of day, this routine will leave you feeling energized or relaxed.

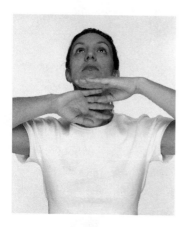

1   Look up to stretch your neck. Using the back of both hands, sweep upwards all the way around the front of the neck for about half a minute. This tones the region.

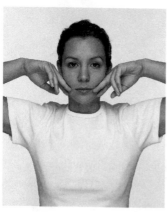

2   From the jawbone, sweep upwards with the back of your index and middle fingers towards the temporal mandibular joint (TMJ) which is by the ear. Repeat on the other side of your face. Hold the skin at this joint for 10 seconds. Repeat five times and then move on to the other side of the face. This helps to reduce any bagginess developing around the jaw line.

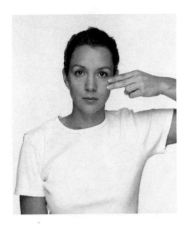

3   Using the pads of the index and middle finger of your left hand, on the left side of the face, gently sweep from the top of the bridge of your nose across the cheeks and up to the top of the ears. Hold for 10 seconds. Repeat on the other side. This helps to lift the cheeks.

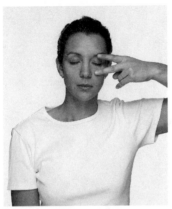

4   Make a V shape with your index and middle fingers. Close your eyes. Place your index finger just below the eyebrow and your middle finger below the eye itself. Use the pads of the fingers to gently sweep across the eye. Continue the movement into the hairline and hold. This helps to reduce bags. Repeat five times.

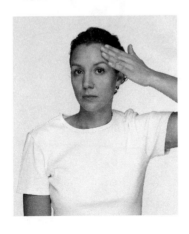

5   Using 3 or 4 fingers, depending on the width of your forehead, gently sweep up your forehead into the hairline. Begin at one temple and continue across to the other temple. This helps to reduce lines across your forehead.

case study

Name: Shirley

Age: 25

Occupation: Interior designer

Shirley came for treatment because she felt that the area under her eyes needed some attention. On her first visit she was shown her face in the mirror halfway through the treatment to compare the side that had been worked on with the one that hadn't – and even with such a small amount of work she could see a big difference.

Since her initial course of treatment, Shirley has a face lift massage once a month, and particularly loves the relaxation part of the treatment. She closes her eyes and within minutes falls asleep. Upon waking she feels wonderful and claims it's better than eight hours of sleep!

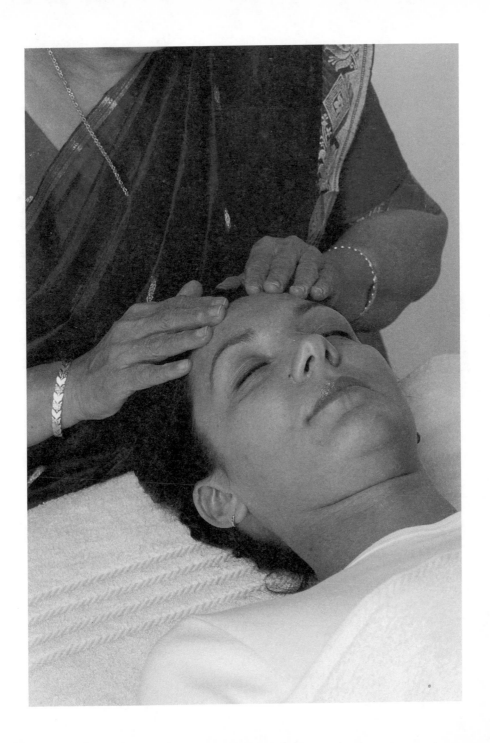

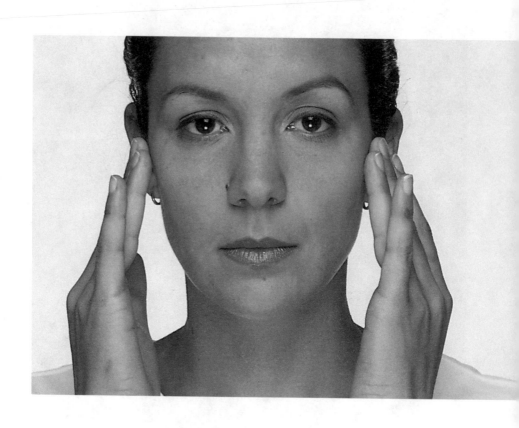

face lift massage

a hands-on experience

Massaging yourself is highly beneficial, but having someone else do it is even more magical. If you are given a weekly facial massage by a partner or therapist, for example, you'll notice a difference after just a few sessions. You won't believe how relaxed, stress-free, and at ease with the world you'll feel after someone has massaged your face.

As if that's not enough, you'll actually see the wrinkles diminish and your face will feel lifted. This is the basis of face lift massage. You should keep up with your own self-help exercises, too, as these will help to consolidate the progress you make. Bear in mind that while you'll see pleasing results from a massage performed at home, you should also experience a massage from a professional who has trained in the technique. With expert help, you can usually see a difference after just one session.

how does face lift massage work?

Face lift massage is a gentle, non-invasive approach to looking younger. Although it's impossible to fend off the aging process altogether, there is much you can do to extend the appearance of youth by means of simple, natural, and effective techniques that make the most of the assets you possess. The light and gentle touch that is used in face lift massage helps to relax the muscles, acts on the connective tissue to untangle and mobilize the fibers, and encourages the ground substance to loosen up and become more fluid.

In face lift massage, we work towards reversing the aging process by releasing the face from any ingrained expressions, freeing constrictions and helping to restore vitality and mobility to the face, thus giving the muscles a new lease of life. This is a precise healthcare system that works the face systematically: releasing deep-seated tensions, freeing layers of muscle and connective tissue so the muscles have space to relax, and encouraging the tissues to glide more smoothly over the deeper layers of muscle and bone.

before and after

It is a good idea to take a couple of close-up photographs of your massage partner's face from different angles before you begin the sessions. You can then take a photograph after the fourth session to see how well things are progressing and another picture at the end of a course of eight to ten sessions to judge the results. While the sessions themselves will feel wonderful and her skin

Identifying problem areas

If you are working on a partner or friend, the first step is to take a close look at her or his facial structure to recognize any problem areas. Please note that this massage is equally suitable for men and women. Make a note or, if you are feeling artistic, sketch out the areas that need most attention.

- **Skin type:** Is the skin normal, dry, oily or combination (oily around the nose and forehead and dry elsewhere)?
- **Skin tone:** Is the skin mainly firm or sagging?
- **Symmetry:** Few faces are truly symmetrical but we are mainly concerned here with lines caused by ingrained expressions and wrinkles.
- **Puffiness:** This can indicate a blockage restricting the flow of lymph and is usually most noticeable around the eyes and jaw line.
- **Expressiveness:** A mask-like quality indicates deep-seated muscular tensions. An expressive face shows the muscles are mobile and supple.
- **Lines or wrinkles:** These areas need extra attention and may also be a sign of other problems.
- **Restrictions:** Some areas may look as if something is preventing them moving freely. This is due to restrictions in the connective tissue.
- **Special areas:** Make a note of scars, injuries or other special problems.
- **Massage partner's priorities:** Your partner's opinion may be different from yours so ask which areas she specifically wants you to tackle.

will be smoother and more toned, it's difficult for someone to appreciate the overall effect of the treatments unless she can make a comparison. By having pictures to compare, she'll be able to see for herself the definite changes in skin tone and structure.

the right mental approach

This form of therapy beautifully combines physical massage and chakra energy balancing techniques. The recipient surrenders her body to the therapist. She suspends her defense mechanisms and, in receiving the massage, is effectively allowing her energy to be balanced. This means she's on a lower energy platform. Recipients must be mentally fully prepared to accept the massage because if they put up any resistance, perhaps by remaining self-conscious and not allowing themselves to relax completely, they will not obtain the maximum benefits. The therapist must be physically and mentally balanced as this greatly increases the likelihood that the treatment will be effective.

Practitioners of Ayurveda believe that energy flows from a higher level to a lower one. This certainly applies when one is being massaged. Therapists are automatically on the higher level for they are channeling the energy through the massage, helping the receiver to rebalance her energy fields. Pulses of pure energy pass from the therapist's fingertips to the skin of the recipient, where it is absorbed, thereby transferring energy from the giver to the receiver.

According to ancient Indian tradition, when you touch someone whatever you are thinking or feeling is transferred to them. So it is important to clear your mind of any impure thoughts or negative feelings beforehand – as this could be passed on through your touch – and set your mind on a higher plain. Spend a few minutes relaxing and meditating, filling yourself with wonderful, healing thoughts before you start the massage. When you are ready and feel in a healing frame of mind, you are ready to give a massage.

Preparing yourself

If you follow these steps you'll be physically and mentally prepared, feeling positive and thinking clearly, and confident you can perform the massage to the best of your ability.

❀ Begin by finding a comfortable position to sit in, with your back straight.

❀ Tuck your chin in a little. You'll find this releases any strain you may have in your neck.

❀ Place your tongue behind your front teeth and concentrate as you breathe in and out, slowly and deeply through your nose, keeping your mouth closed.

❀ Bend your elbows and bring your hands up to the level of your heart. Meanwhile let your shoulders drop as they relax.

❀ Cup your hands in front of you and imagine they are being filled with a ball of healing energy. Imagine this energy is being passed through your hands to your heart. Notice how strong and full of positive energy you feel.

❀ Rub the backs of your hands together and then the palms to create energy and warmth.

❀ Direct your mind towards your massage partner with healing thoughts.

the magic of massage

For the massage to be most effective, your massage partner must feel he or she can trust you and feel confident and comfortable in your hands. So it is important to encourage your partner to feel more open to the experience. After the massage, both the therapist and the receiver should have a brief rest to gather and rebalance their energies.

stage 1: relaxation and exploration

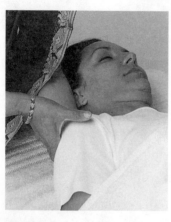

Ask your massage partner to lie down. Place a blanket over her to keep her warm. When she is comfortable, encourage her to relax by slipping a hand under her right shoulder blade. Ask her to breathe in and then breathe out, sliding your hand out as she exhales. This helps her to breathe freely and to let go of any tension she may be holding in her shoulders, making it easier for you to work. Repeat the move, this time placing your hand under her left shoulder blade. Now check to see if she is breathing easily. Be warned – she may be so relaxed that she falls asleep!

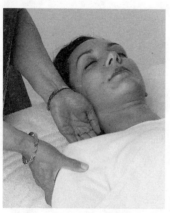

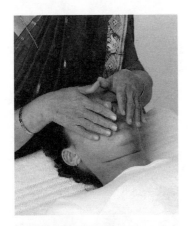

You are about to use energy balancing. Place both hands 3 in (7.5 cm) above your partner's face, transferring the universal energy to calm her and relax her further. Breathe deeply and slowly. With each breath bring your hands closer to your partner's face until you gently make contact with the skin.

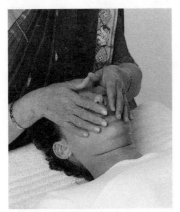

Lay your hands on her face and hold them there for a few seconds. This helps you to ground yourself and allows your partner to relax her face.

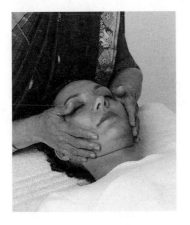

Slide your hands out until they are above her ears and hold them there for a few seconds.

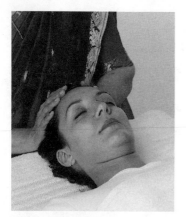

Move your hands and place them over her head at the crown chakra. This helps to balance your partner's energy. Hold your hands there for 30 seconds. The whole process should take 2–3 minutes.

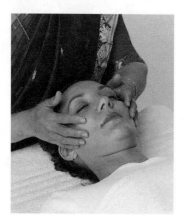

Stroke the sides of your partner's face three times, using light, gentle pressure. This will soothe her nervous system, relaxing her even more.

These exercises are designed to stimulate Ayurvedic pressure points. In each case apply gentle pressure and hold each pressure point for 10 seconds.

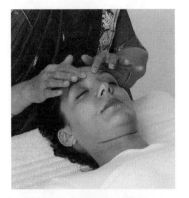

With the pads of both index or middle fingers, gently press down at the top of the eyebrows to lightly stimulate the pressure points. Continue these movements in the middle of the forehead, gradually working up towards the hairline, breaking down restricted tissue. Carry on, working the forehead in parallel strips. Hold each pressure point for about 10 seconds.

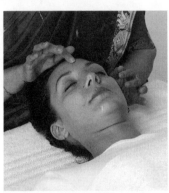

Place light pressure on the middle of the forehead with the index finger of your right hand.

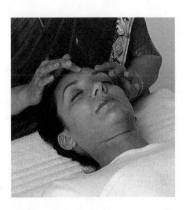

While still applying pressure here, use your index finger to apply pressure about 1 in (2.5 cm) to the left of the third eye. Repeat with the right hand.

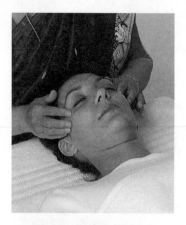

Now stimulate the pressure points on the outer corners of both eyes.

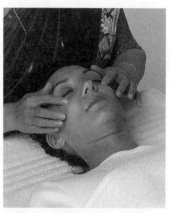

Now stimulate the pressure points below the eyes, holding for about 10 seconds.

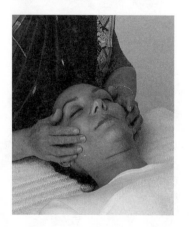

Find the cheek pressure points, which are about 1 in (2.5 cm) away from the corners of the mouth and parallel to each corner. Apply gentle pressure to each one for 10 seconds.

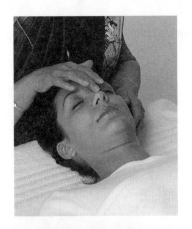

Using the index or middle finger of your dominant hand, apply gentle pressure to the tip of the nose.

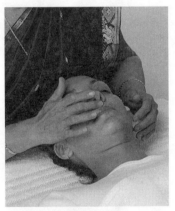

Move to the point between the nose and the middle of the upper lip, and apply gentle pressure here for 10 seconds.

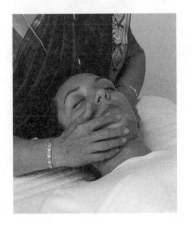

Move your finger to the center of the chin and apply pressure here.

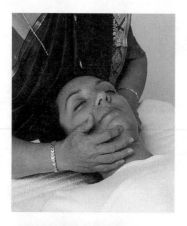

Now slip your finger down to below the center of the chin and apply pressure.

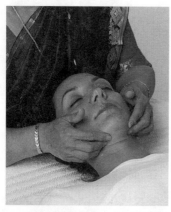

Using your index fingers, stimulate the pressure points on the jaw line.

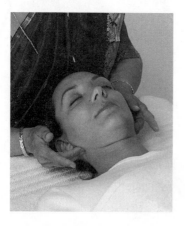

Change to your middle finger, for ease, and work the points below the ears.

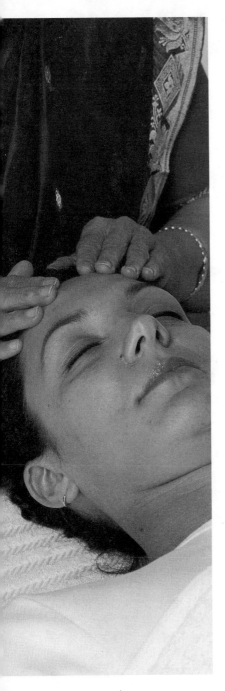

stage 3: initial releases

You have successfully passed through the first two stages of this process. Take a few seconds to relax and prepare before moving on to stage 3. Now you're ready to begin the main phase, starting off with initial releases. Initial releases are done all over the face using the pads of three fingers of both hands, moving them in a circular manner. You start by massaging the surface of the skin, gradually making your strokes deeper to allow the muscles to become more mobile. You should be aware of the fact that when you work on these muscles repressed emotions may be released (people have been known to cry) so be prepared for the unexpected.

Begin on the middle of the forehead and work your way out and down on either side of the eyes. Now move below the eyes and over the cheeks towards the nose, then out towards the ears, back to the mouth, over the chin and out towards the jaw, finally moving below the chin. Work in a zigzag manner, gradually moving down the face. Remember, initially use quite light pressure, as you only want to make an impact at surface level. Then repeat this whole movement with slightly more pressure to make the muscles more mobile and release more tension. Now the recipient is prepared for the benefits that stage 4 has to offer.

stage 4: smoothing out the tension

These steps will not only leave the recipient feeling incredibly relaxed, they're also effective at releasing any tension that has built up in the face. Spend about ten minutes gently working the face, discovering where the skin and muscles are constricted, and then take some time to very gently release blocked connective tissue. You are looking for micro movements under the mound at the base of the thumb that show that the restrictions are slowly being released. Working around wrinkles releasing the connective tissue is amazingly effective at reducing their prominence. When you come across constricted tissue, keep your movements small and move into the resistance to loosen it. Work in a variety of directions to maximize the release. As you work, take care to avoid stretching the skin.

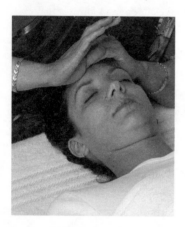

Use the mound at the base of the thumb of your right hand for the right side of the recipient's face. When you work on the left side of the recipient's face, use the mound at the base of the thumb on your left hand. Working on the right side of the face first, begin in the middle of the forehead. Hold an area of skin with the forefinger of your left hand. Let the base of your right thumb glide past and around your forefinger in a semi-circular movement, as you lightly twist your wrist. Follow the route given in Stage 5 over the right side of the recipient's face and then swap hands and work on the left side of their face.

stage 5: stabilizing

Concentrate on working on one half of the face at a time. Start with the side that you think needs most attention. Using the index finger of one hand as a stabilizing or mother finger, use the index finger of the other hand to slide around the mother finger in a semi-circular movement. For example, if you decide to work on the right side of the face, use the index finger of your left hand as the stabilizing or mother finger. Gently slide the index finger of the right hand around the left index finger in an inward direction. Then exert a gentle lifting action (i.e. gently coaxing the skin in an upwards direction towards you) using the pads of the fingers. This is one complete movement. Take the route described in the following pictures.

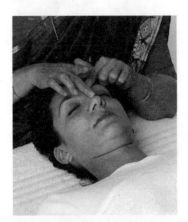

Starting between the eyebrows, gently work down the nose from the bridge to the tip and back up again, using gentle sliding movements. This is an important step because there is usually a great deal of tension (and often wrinkles) in this area.

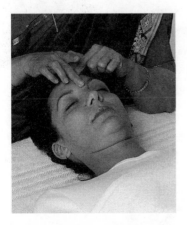

Return to the forehead and begin working your way up to the hairline with a gentle sliding action combined with gentle downward movements, allowing tension in the tissues to be released.

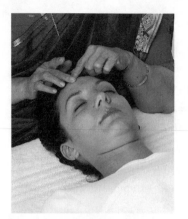

Repeat these movements in a zigzag fashion from the eyebrow to the hairline and back again, covering the whole of that half of the forehead. Now work horizontally, still covering the same half of the forehead.

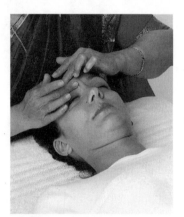

Work your way slowly up to the temples and place one finger just above the eyebrow. Then slide upwards and outwards across the eyebrow in a crosswise movement that helps to break up tension and restrictions in the tissues. Keep the pressure even and continuous. If you come across any particular lines don't try to work on them specifically.

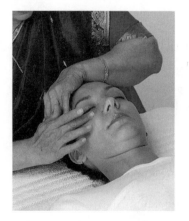

Move on to the area below the eyebrow ridge. Using a slow movement, continue around the sides of the eyes and then work the eye muscle, at the same time using the mother finger to stabilize the skin just underneath.

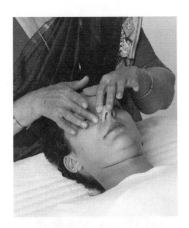

Work the side of the bridge of the nose, still with one finger serving as a mother finger.

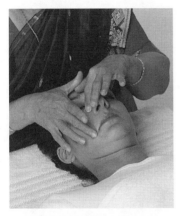

Now move down towards the corner of the mouth.

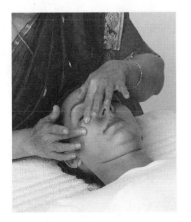

Work across the cheeks from top to bottom, moving towards the lips in a diagonal movement, one finger holding down, continually looking for restrictions. Slide down and across

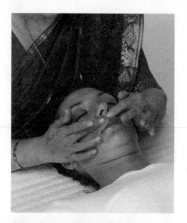

Now work around the mouth. The distance between the two fingers around should be about 1 in (2.5 cm), with one remaining static below the middle of the nose and the other pushing the upper lip towards the other finger. The mouth is used a lot, so there could be many restrictions here.

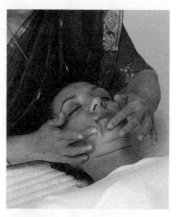

Using the same technique, with one finger acting as the mother finger, work the corner of the mouth. Work your way down to the chin and then underneath, releasing tension in this area. Continue to work all the way down to the side of the neck.

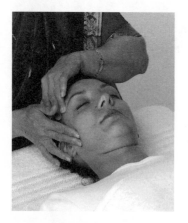

Use a couple of fingers to hold the temples and, moving in tandem with the other hand, sweep down using a traction movement to encourage the circulation.

stage 6: deeper releases using the healing pulse

The healing pulse is felt as a throbbing at various points on the face and neck. As the name suggests, stimulating the healing pulse has many therapeutic benefits.

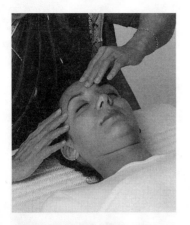

Place two fingers of one hand by the temples and, with the other hand, place the index finger in the middle of the forehead and the middle finger between the eyebrows at the top of the nose. Gently hold the area until you can feel the throbbing of the healing pulse, then release. Work your way inwards using the same movements until the fingers of both hands meet. If the temple is very wide, repeat these movements higher up.

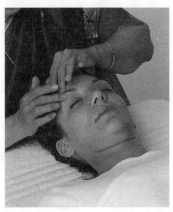

Place the index finger of the left hand above the eyebrow and prepare to push down gently. Now place the middle finger of the right hand below the eyebrow and diagonally across. Once both fingers are in place, push upwards and downwards creating a traction or tightness in the area. Hold this position until you feel the healing pulse.

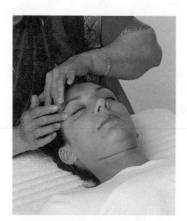

Use the healing pulse around the eyes by creating a tiny space between two fingers at the top and bottom of the eyebrow to release tension there. Choose which fingers feel the most comfortable for this.

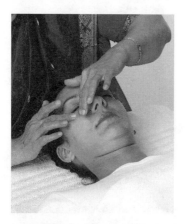

Use the same technique at the bottom of the eye muscle. Start at the inner corner and gradually work towards the middle and then the far side.

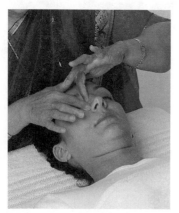

Work the side of the nose in the same way and then a little further down. This stimulates the flow of lymph. Now place the left hand at the side of the cheek and, using the right hand, pull up about 2 in (5 cm) from the corner of the mouth. This releases tension.

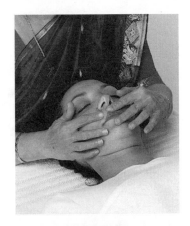

Move on to the lips, then below the lips, outwards across the jaw line, and then in front of the ears. Hold each position until you feel the throbbing of the healing pulse. Don't worry if you cannot feel any pulsations on your first attempt – with practice you will!

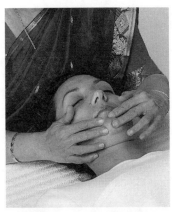

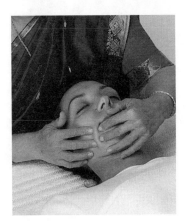

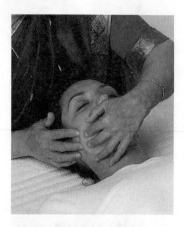

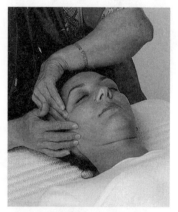

Use the same manoeuvre in the temple area.

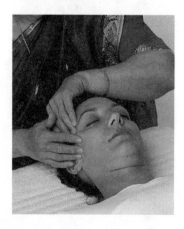

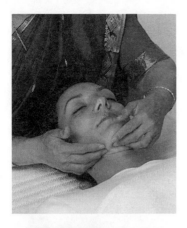

Work right under the chin, pressing the flesh slightly, working to the end of the chin.

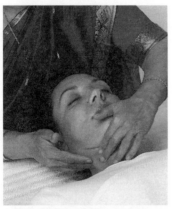

Using a couple of fingers, grasp the skin below the chin and press down and pull upwards by the sternocleidomastoid muscle. This releases restrictions and improves circulation and energy flow throughout the face.

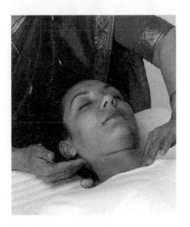

Place one finger on the sternum and your right hand behind the earlobe and press down. This too releases tension.

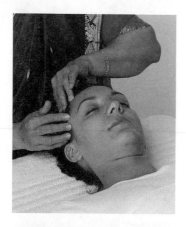

Use the healing pulse at the hairline to release tension in the scalp. Then apply the pressure to the scalp and temples.

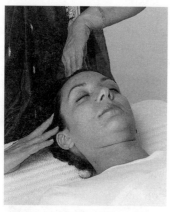

Use the healing pulse just above the ear and middle of the skull and slowly move your hands closer together until the fingers meet.

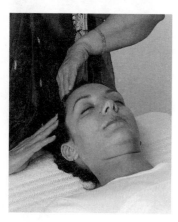

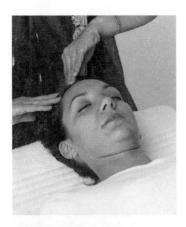

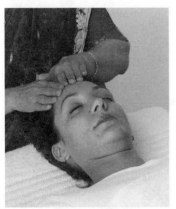

Stroke up towards the forehead and hairline,
working both upwards and outwards.

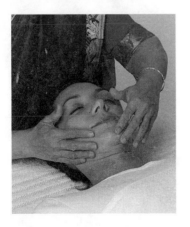

Now use one hand as a mother hand and stroke
upwards all over the face with the other.

Let your massage partner get up to have a look at the work you've done so far. It is important to do it at this stage, before you start on the other side of the face, so she can see the differences between the two sides. She'll probably tell you how stiff and dull the other side of the face feels.

Now repeat stages 5 and 6, this time working the other side of the face. When you have worked both sides of the face, perform the following two steps.

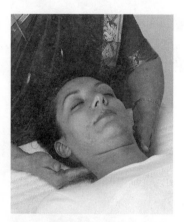

Hold both sides of the top of her neck for a few seconds.

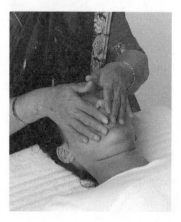

Now move your hands over her face and hold lightly for a few seconds to give healing and warmth.

stage 8: grounding

When the session is over it's important to ground your partner so she can carry on in an alert and centered fashion. Your massage partner has been lying down for up to an hour by now, so this exercise is important to get her energy moving.

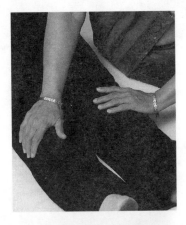

Proceed with energy balancing by gently squeezing both thighs.

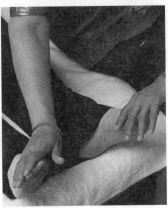

Work down her legs and then gently squeeze her feet and toes. Now sweep down her thighs, legs, feet, and toes with your fingertips. Do this three times.

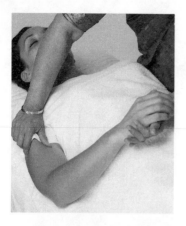

Repeat the energy balancing with her arms and hands.

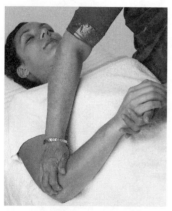

Now knead her upper forearms and rub her hands one after the other.

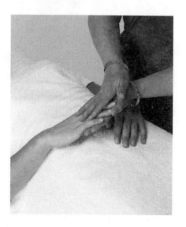

Finally, gently sweep down from her shoulder to the tips of her fingers, one arm at a time. Perform this move three times on each arm.

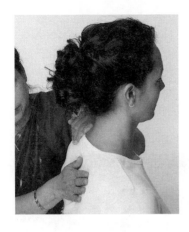

You may have to help her sit up and then rub her shoulders and back. Then using your fingertips gently sweep down three times from the crown of her head to her lower back to help your partner ground herself.

It's a good idea for both you and your partner to enjoy a refreshing glass of pure water once the treatment is over. They'll probably tell you they feel fantastic! Thanks to you, they'll be looking great too!

Kundun Mehta, the author of this book, runs training courses worldwide in this wonderful therapy. For details of a Face Lift Massage (Facial Rejuvenation) training course near you, contact her at:

London Centre of Indian Champissage International
136 Holloway Road
London N7 8DD
Tel: (+44) 207 609 3590

You can send an email to mehta@indianchampissage.com
or visit the website at www.indianchampissage.com

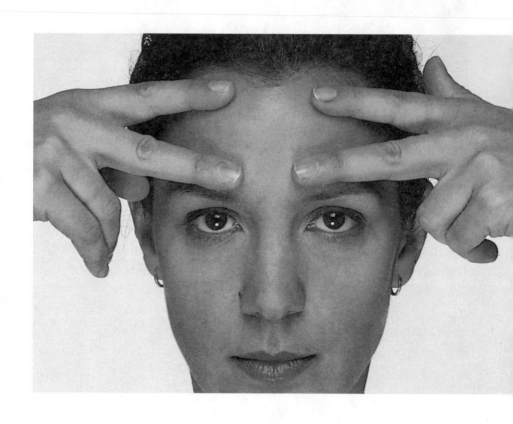

recipes for natural beauty

feeding the outer self

There's no big secret to having healthy, young-looking skin. Simple routines using natural products can produce stunning results. What's more, a little pampering from time to time not only nourishes your skin but also gives you time to focus on yourself and wind down from the stresses and strains of modern life. It is vital to nourish your skin from inside, too and we shall be looking at the importance of healthy eating in Chapter 7, but you should also maintain a regular skincare routine.

In a quest for youthful-looking skin, many people spend a lot of money on skincare products. But this is not an ideal solution. Shop-bought items can be expensive, are not necessarily effective, and can also cause problems of their own, such as clogged pores, spots, skin-sensitivity disorders and allergies. You don't have to pay a fortune to take care of your skin. For thousands of years, women have looked to nature to find the answers to their skin problems with great success.

In India it was always considered perfectly normal to design your own beauty regime and to make beauty products using natural ingredients. But more recently people have been swept along by a tide of mass-produced creams and lotions manufactured by the large cosmetic companies and as a result they almost forgot the traditions of their ancestors. Now there is a huge resurgence of interest in the traditional approach, and it is catching on in the West, too. In this chapter we'll show you how to make yourself beautiful with natural ingredients, many of which can be found in your own home.

The benefits of natural skincare are many and various. You decide what to put on your skin, and you spend far less on ingredients than you would on shop-bought products. You'll find the process of making beauty products relaxing in itself. It enables you to focus on yourself and to switch off the decision-making left-hand side of your brain, allowing the more creative right-hand side to take over.

Nature provides you with all the cleansers, toners, astringents, and face packs you could possibly need. If you look in your kitchen cupboard and refrigerator you may be surprised to find that you already have many of the core ingredients that will keep your skin looking healthy and supple, and which can naturally help to fight the ravages of time. Recent studies show that when certain vitamins and minerals are put straight on to the skin they can actually reverse some of the damage caused by sun, pollution, and stress. These are the so-called antioxidants, which include vitamins A, C, and E, the plant pigment beta-carotene (which is converted to vitamin A in the body), and the minerals zinc and selenium. When applied to the face, they counteract the damaging effect of free radicals (see Glossary), a major cause of skin aging. Vitamin C also stimulates tissue regeneration.

First we will look at some natural ingredients and explain what they can do.
Later we will explain how to combine them to make all the natural beauty
products you could need. Where possible, always choose organic products, which
are free of potentially harmful additives. However, as natural skincare products
do not contain preservatives, they won't last as long as manufactured kinds. All
natural products must be stored in the refrigerator and most should be kept for
no longer than a few days. If you plan to keep these products in jars or other
containers, always sterilize them first using boiling water.

❀ *Yogurt: This contains lactic acid which draws oil and bacteria out of the pores while
pulling moisture in. It smoothes, moisturizes, tightens, and tones the skin and is ideal
for those with oily, spotty skin. It can be applied straight on to the face without
adding any other ingredients. Leave on the skin for 20 minutes and then rinse off
with lukewarm water.*

❀ *Honey: This is a natural moisturizer. It hydrates the skin and helps many dry skin
conditions. It also has mildly antiseptic qualities, so it is highly beneficial for oily skin
that is prone to spots. Used on its own and applied directly to the face, it leaves the
skin with a soft, satiny look.*

❀ *Egg: Both the white and yolk of the egg are beneficial. The white closes the pores
and tones the skin while the yolk is a natural moisturizer. They can be used
separately in various products or you can take a whole egg, whip it up, and apply it
directly to your skin. Leave it on for a few minutes and then rinse off. You'll notice
your skin tightens and lifts.*

❀ *Turmeric: This is traditionally used in India to beautify a bride before her wedding
day. It has antiseptic qualities, which clear the complexion, and also softens the skin.
When combined with other ingredients in a face mask, it leaves the skin with an
amazing glow.*

- **✿ Flour:** *Certain types of flour can nourish and cleanse the skin. In India, gram flour is still used as a cleanser when mixed with a little milk and applied to the face. It is also used as a base for many other beauty products.*

- **✿ Brewer's yeast:** *This makes an effective cleanser when combined with other ingredients and is particularly beneficial for oily skin.*

- **✿ Olive oil:** *This can soften, moisturize, and soothe the skin. Always choose organic oils, which are produced without the use of chemical fertilizers or pesticides.*

- **✿ Rosewater:** *This is a byproduct of the distillation of the essential oil of roses. It is slightly acidic so it acts as a good toner, promoting regeneration, tightening the skin, and counteracting infection. Orange water is better suited to oily skin.*

- **✿ Sugar:** *When rubbed on to the skin, sugar acts as an exfoliant to remove dead cells and so brighten the skin. It can also counteract infection.*

- **✿ Oatmeal:** *This soothes, lightens, and exfoliates the skin. It is also a natural source of vitamin E, one of the antioxidant vitamins that help counteract the damaging effect of free radicals in the skin.*

fruit and vegetables – wonder ingredients

As well as being high in antioxidants, many fruits and vegetables are rich in enzymes that leave your face feeling toned, tingling, and glowing. When you make your own face products at home they contain far more nutrients than anything you can buy in the shops. There are certain combinations of fruit and vegetable that are best for particular skin types.

oily skin

✿ **Apricot:** *Many skin products sold in shops contain apricot, for a very good reason. Apricot is a rich source of plant chemicals called beta-carotenes, which are powerful antioxidants. They are also converted in the body into the antioxidant vitamin A, which is needed for healthy skin and has a rejuvenating effect on the face, helping to smooth away wrinkles and lighten stretch marks. Apricot also contains enzymes that act as a strong antiseptic and astringent.*

✿ **Cucumber:** *This is a skin refresher. Slicing cucumber and placing it over the eyes has become a popular home treatment for tired or puffy eyes but it is also of great benefit to other parts of the face as it is a natural astringent and helps to close pores. After a hot and sticky day, wipe your skin with slices of cucumber and you'll feel how refreshing it can be.*

✿ **Eucalyptus:** *This has natural antiseptic qualities and soothes, heals, and refreshes the skin.*

✿ **Lemon:** *This is a natural astringent and helps to neutralize bacteria, close pores, fade blemishes, and eradicate spots. It is a rich source of vitamin C, an antioxidant and an important vitamin for skin repair and renewal.*

dry skin

✿ **Avocado:** *Dry skin needs to be pumped up with moisture and avocado is ideal for this purpose. It is rich in monounsaturated oils which are easily absorbed into the skin. It also contains vitamin E.*

✿ **Banana:** *Mashed banana is effective at hydrating the skin.*

✿ **Carrot:** *This soothes dry, sensitive skin and is a good source of carotenes, which are antioxidants, and in particular beta-carotenes, which are converted into vitamin A in the body.*

❀ **Comfrey:** *Oils extracted from this herb are very good for dehydrated skin.*

❀ **Grape:** *This is rich in trace elements that are thought to aid the regeneration of new skin cells.*

❀ **Papaya:** *The pulp of the papaya contains an enzyme that removes dead skin cells when applied to the face. It is also a rich source of antioxidants such as beta-carotenes and vitamin C.*

❀ **Potato:** *This helps to clear skin blemishes and can be beneficial in cases of eczema. Potato slices placed over the eyes can reduce bagginess.*

❀ **Rose:** *Petals taken from fresh rose flowers and soaked in spring water make an ideal base for skin tonics that soothe rough skin.*

normal skin

❀ **Almond:** *This is one of the most effective beauty ingredients for normal skin. It acts as a moisturizer but also tightens the skin.*

❀ **Peach:** *This is soothing and acts as a mild lubricant.*

Understanding your skin type

Before you start a skincare program, it is important to identify the type of skin you have. Bear in mind that the condition of the skin changes week by week and month by month and can alter dramatically over the course of a lifetime, so be prepared to vary your routine to match your current complexion. For instance, the skin produces more sebum at certain times of the month, and this will affect the oiliness of the skin.

Before you wash your face in the morning, press a large open tissue against your face, holding it in place for a few moments. Now hold the tissue up to the light. If it is completely clean, your skin is dry and possibly sensitive. If there is a trace of sebum, your skin is normal. If there is a clear T-shaped imprint of sebum from the nose and forehead you have combination skin. A complete print of your face is a sign of oily skin.

cleansing and moisturizing

The keys to an effective skincare routine are thorough cleansing and regular moisturizing, although they can't completely undo damage caused by excessive exposure to the sun or years of poor diet. Soap is not regarded as part of a beauty treatment in India and is rarely used on the face because of its drying effect. It is highly alkaline and can damage the skin's natural protective film, the acid mantle. Soap can't cleanse the pores thoroughly enough to prevent spots and blackheads. Alcohol is found in many beauty products, but is best avoided as, like soap, it has a serious drying effect. For most skins, an oil-based cleanser is best, used mornings and evenings.

All skin types need moisturizer, even oily skins. Moisturizer improves the appearance of the outer, cornified, layer, making it feel smoother and softer, and provides a physical barrier to protect skin from the elements and guard against bacterial invasion. Moisturizer also helps keep the skin hydrated and prevents dry air from pulling moisture out of the skin. Moisturizer should be porous to allow the skin to breathe.

Only moisture from within can really improve the skin's appearance over a longer period, however. Many manufactured products contain glycerine, which draws the skin's moisture to the surface. But it is only effective if there is enough water in the rest of the body to keep the skin moist and to replace what is lost. Water sprays or spritzers are useful for topping up moisture levels in the skin throughout the day, especially if you live or work in an environment made as arid as a desert by central heating or air conditioning.

dry and mature skin

This skin type is prone to premature aging. Mature skin loses moisture more rapidly as the natural oil barrier breaks down with age. Skin dryness is mainly caused by lack of water in the paper-thin, non-living top layers of skin. Despite what advertisers claim, only the top layers of the skin need moisturizing. Be wary of creams that claim to moisturize the deepest layers of the skin as dryness does not usually affect this region. Signs of aging due to dry skin probably won't show up until you are in your fifties. Most wrinkling that appears before this is due to sun damage.

cleansing

To help preserve the protective oily film, the acid mantle, which covers the skin and locks in moisture, avoid soap and water. If you prefer, wash off cleansers using a soap-free bar or face wash, but restrict this to the mornings. Constantly wetting and drying the skin makes a dry-skin condition worse. It is better to use a cream or oil-based cleanser in the morning and evening. Apply a little to the skin, massage in gently, leave for a few seconds, then wipe off with cotton wool, a damp flannel or a soft muslin cloth. Damp cotton wool is ideal as it stops moisture being drawn out of the skin. Tissues are best avoided as they can scratch delicate skin. Cactus has an incredibly high moisture retention capacity and is ideal for rehydrating the skin, so try to find a cleanser that contains this ingredient. If you use a toner make sure it is alcohol-free.

You may wish to make your own cleanser. You can experiment with various types of natural products that you think may suit your skin type but here are a couple of examples of cleansers that can be made at home.

almond and honey cleanser

This recipe combines the moisturizing benefits of almond with the cleansing nature of honey.

INGREDIENTS:

3 tsp honey

6 tbsp almonds that have been brought to boiling in water, cooled, and skinned

¾ cup (150 ml) mineral water

4 tbsp rosewater

METHOD:

In a blender, mix together the honey, almonds, and mineral water and leave the mixture overnight in the refrigerator. Place the mixture in the center of a clean muslin cloth. Bring the edges of the cloth together, place over a bowl and squeeze the cloth to strain out the juice. Discard the contents of the cloth. Finally, add the rosewater to the extracted juice. Apply this to the face with cotton wool and wash it off with lukewarm water. This mixture can last up to two weeks in a refrigerator.

natural-oil cleanser

This recipe will suit those who prefer to use an oil-based cleanser.

INGREDIENTS:

5 tbsp sesame oil

A few drops each of sandalwood, geranium, and rose essential oils

4 tbsp aloe vera juice

1 tbsp almond oil

1 tbsp avocado oil

1 tbsp glycerine

1 tbsp jojoba oil

1 tbsp sunflower oil

1 tbsp vitamin E oil

METHOD:

Mix all the ingredients together and pour into a bottle with a tight-fitting lid. Shake the bottle to bring the mixture to the right constituency. Apply to the face using circular movements and then remove using a damp muslin cloth or damp cotton wool.

moisturizing

Dry and mature skin needs more regular moisturizing than younger skin. It is best to apply a moisturizer directly after cleansing. Over time you will notice that your skin doesn't produce as much natural oil as it used to, which reduces its ability to retain moisture. This can leave the face looking wrinkled and feeling dry, rough, and less flexible. Applying moisturizer can help to prevent this. Choose one that is absorbed easily and doesn't leave a greasy film on the skin. Top up moisture levels throughout the day by spritzing your skin frequently with a water spray or spray-on tonic. If your skin is very dry and you live in a centrally heated home, consider using a humidifier to put moisture back into the air. Try the following moisturizer:

aloe vera moisturizer

INGREDIENTS:

⅓ cup (75 ml) sesame oil for dry skin or
rice bran oil or ghee for mature skin
⅛ cup (25 ml) cocoa butter or lanolin
¼ cup (50 ml) rosewater
2 tbsp aloe vera gel

METHOD:

Warm the oils and butter together; warm the rosewater and aloe vera gel separately. Place all the ingredients in a blender and mix. Transfer the mixture to a container. Let the mixture cool. Apply to the skin as necessary.

combination skin

This is a very common skin type, even in older women. Oily areas on the forehead, nose, and chin may be made worse by hormonal factors or a diet that is too high in saturated fats. Dry cheeks are often a consequence of living in dry conditions, usually due to central heating or air conditioning. Many people mistake dry, flaky patches on the nose and forehead as dry skin. In fact, this is the result of excessive sebum production. Too much moisturizing and not enough cleansing can cause the skin condition seborrhoeic dermatitis. This causes the top layer of skin to flake off.

cleansing

To prevent spots and blackheads, which often appear in oily areas, cleanse twice a day with a soap-free or oil-based cleanser. Oil-based cleansers work well on oily areas of skin as they dissolve the skin's own sebum and gently remove any excess. You can use the recipe on page 122 for oily skin. It's not essential to use a toner but may help to reduce the number of large pores.

moisturizing

After cleansing, apply moisturizer twice daily all over your face, not just on the dry areas, as the dehydration that leads to wrinkling is not caused by oil on the skin but by a lack of water in the top layers. The sebum on your skin serves to trap the moisture below this layer.

oily skin

Cleansing is one of the most important daily rituals for oily skin. But don't overdo it. Proper cleansing is essential to prevent pores getting clogged, but excessive cleansing can cause the skin to produce even more sebum, so try to strike a happy medium. Unfortunately, excess oil on the face traps dirt and over the course of the day the skin can be covered with a fine layer of grime. If you need proof, at the end of the day gently drag one of your finger nails across your forehead or cheek and you'll see the dirt collect under your nail! It is important to remove this each day or your skin will soon be covered in blackheads and spots. Some people say you should not moisturize if you have oily skin as it can make the problem worse, but this is not true. As with all types of skin, you just need to be careful about the type of moisturizer you choose.

cleansing

Oily skin often looks shiny and has enlarged pores, giving it a thick appearance, due to the excess secretion of sebum. If you don't maintain a thorough cleansing routine, these pores not only hold grease and dirt but also stale sweat and make-up, which can lead to other skin problems. If you have a very oily diet this also shows itself on your face. If you use a soap-free facial wash follow this with an oil-based cleanser, since sebum dissolves in oil and not water. Apply to the skin twice daily, massaging well in, and then remove with damp cotton wool. You could also use a toner made from rosewater to remove any final traces of dirt. If you suffer from spots or acne try tea tree oil. This has drying and antiseptic properties without leaving behind a flaky surface. Here are two recipes for cleansers for oily skin:

jojoba cleanser

INGREDIENTS:

5 tbsp jojoba oil
A few drops of lemon and cypress essential oils
4 tbsp aloe vera juice
1 tbsp almond oil
1 tbsp glycerine
1 tbsp sunflower oil
1 tbsp vitamin E oil

METHOD:

Mix the ingredients and pour into a bottle with a tight-fitting lid. Shake well. Apply to the face in circular movements and then remove with a moist muslin cloth or damp cotton wool.

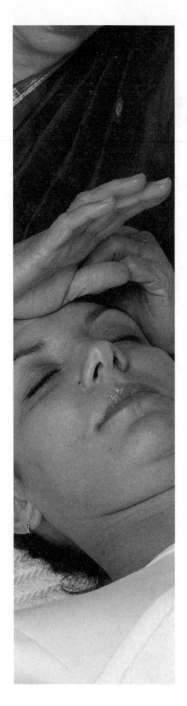

herbal cleanser

INGREDIENTS:

4 heaped tbsp of freshly chopped lemon peel, sage,
and mint, mixed
⅔ cup (140 ml) whole milk

METHOD:

Add the fresh herbs and lemon peel to the
cold milk. Cover and soak for four hours in a
cool place. Strain the mixture through a sieve,
using a wooden spoon to press as much liquid
out as you can. Discard the herbs. Apply the
herbalized milk with cotton wool and remove
by splashing with warm water. Keep the
mixture in the refrigerator and use within
four days.

moisturizing

Oily skin needs a moisturizer. Choose a light
moisturizer and apply it after cleansing. Good
quality moisturizers often contain ingredients
such as vitamins, sunscreen, and herbal extracts
that can aid oily complexions.

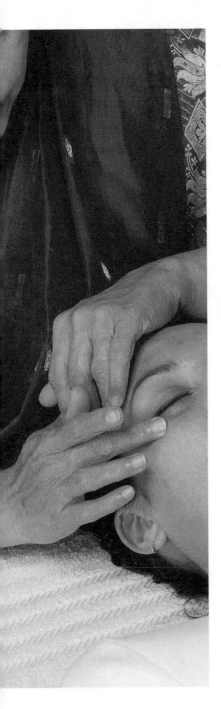

mint and witch hazel moisturizer

This recipe is especially suited to oily skin.

INGREDIENTS:

2 heaped tsp chopped fresh mint

6 tbsp mineral water

2 tbsp witch hazel

¼ cup (50 ml) rosewater

2 tbsp glycerine

METHOD:

Put the mint in a pan and add the water.
Bring to boiling and simmer for 10 minutes.
Cool the mixture and strain through a sieve or
muslin cloth. Discard the mint. Add the witch
hazel, rosewater, and glycerine to the water.
Put the mixture in a container with a tight-
fitting lid and shake before use. Keep the
mixture in the refrigerator and use within
four days.

normal skin

Regular cleansing is necessary even for normal skin. Apply the following cleanser with a soft muslin cloth every morning and rinse with water.

herbal tea cleanser

INGREDIENTS:

2 heaped tsps of fresh rosemary, camomile, and nettle, mixed
boiling water

METHOD:

Put the herbs in a cup and fill with boiling water. Leave until cold and then strain through a sieve. Discard the herbs and transfer the tea to a bottle. Apply the tea with cotton wool. Keep the mixture in the refrigerator and use within four days.

facial treatments

The following facial treatments can be highly beneficial.

steaming

This is one of the oldest methods of cleansing your face. Steaming your face is a wonderful way of easing muscular tension and clearing the mind of clutter. It also cleanses deep into the pores, making the skin more receptive to moisturizers and masks. As well as deep cleansing, the steam helps to moisturize and plump up the skin, reducing fine lines. Steaming is perfect for combination and oily skin types as it removes blackheads and spots by unblocking sebum-clogged pores.

natural steam treatment

INGREDIENTS:

Normal skin: 1 tsp of dried lavender or sage

Dry skin: 1 tsp of camomile and basil

Combination and oily skins: 1 tsp of mint and lemon peel

If you don't want to use herbs then add the following essential oils to the boiling water:

Normal skin: 3 drops lavender, 3 drops mandarin

Dry skin: 3 drops rose, 3 drops camomile

Combination skin: 3 drops lavender, 3 drops cypress

Oily skin: 3 drops lemon, 3 drops eucalyptus

METHOD:

Fill a large bowl with boiled water and add the appropriate herbs or oils. Stir well and allow to infuse for a few minutes. Place a large towel over your head and neck to form a tent and lean over the bowl. Close your eyes and allow the steam to work for 2–3 minutes. Finally, blot your face with a face cloth and spritz it with a fine water spray.

exfoliating the skin

Exfoliants gently rub off the top layer of dead skin cells, and also boost the circulation of the face. This speeds up the rate at which the skin cells are replaced, encouraging clearer, younger-looking skin to form. As you get older it becomes more important to exfoliate as dead skin cells can make wrinkles appear deeper than they really are. Try not to be too vigorous, as the outer skin layer is the first line of defense against attack from sunlight and pollution. Limit exfoliation to no more than once a week.

One method is to use a muslin cloth to buff away flakes of dead skin and dislodge dingy skin cells. You can buy commercial exfoliants or scrubs but many are too harsh. Be careful if using commercial exfoliants containing crushed nuts or apricot pits as they can be highly abrasive and cause microscopic damage to the structure of the skin. Try making your own exfoliants — you can tailor them to your own skin type but the following suit all.

papaya rub

METHOD:

Take one ripe papaya, slice it in half and peel away the skin in large pieces. Rub the inside of the skin over your face and neck, massaging for 1–2 minutes. Rinse with cool water and then dry. This helps to remove dead skin cells and should leave your skin looking and feeling smoother.

Most scrubs are made from a base of whole grain or bean flour with extra ingredients added to suit particular skin types. Don't be tempted to use tissues to wipe off scrubs as they can scratch the skin. Try the following:

oatmeal scrub

This is for dry, dull-looking skin.

INGREDIENTS:

12 tsp granulated sugar
2 tbsp rosewater
1 tbsp medium-ground oatmeal
1 tsp honey

METHOD:

Mix all the ingredients together in a bowl to make a gritty paste. Apply to the skin using gentle, circular movements, concentrating on the nose, chin, and forehead, to remove flakes of dry skin. Rinse well and pat dry.

sea salt

This is for combination skin.

METHOD:
Rub fine granules of sea salt into wet skin and massage lightly. Rinse well and pat dry.

sugar rub

This is for oily or spotty skin. Sugar has an anti-bacterial effect on the skin.

METHOD:
Mix 1 tbsp of granulated white sugar with a few drops of hot water and massage gently over the face and neck. Rinse with cool water and pat dry.

almond scrub

This is for oily skin.

INGREDIENTS:
2 tsp ground almonds
2 tsp fine oatmeal
Orange flower water

METHOD:
Put all the ingredients in a bowl and mix into a smooth paste. Leave to stand for a few minutes. Gently massage into the face using circular movements and then wipe off with a damp muslin cloth. Rinse thoroughly and pat dry with a towel.

apple scrub

This is for normal skin.

INGREDIENTS:
2 tsp cornstarch/cornflour
1 tsp almond oil
2 tsp brown sugar
Enough apple juice to bind the mixture together

METHOD:
Mix all the ingredients in a bowl. Allow to stand for a few minutes and then apply to the face, using circular movements. Wash off and pat the face dry with a towel.

facial masks

Masks are useful for revitalizing the complexion. But that's not all they do. They also nourish the skin by providing vitamins and minerals that help to heal scars, even out color tone, and soothe and moisturize the skin. They cleanse thoroughly by extracting dirt that lies deep in the pores and so help to prevent blackheads and spots, and they can also stimulate the growth of new skin cells. Clay has been used as one of the basics of face masks for thousands of years, since the Pharaohs praised it for its healing properties and beneficial effect on the skin. The ancient Chinese, Greeks, Romans, and the early people of the Indian subcontinent all knew of its wonderful properties and used it both internally and externally.

Clay cleanses deeply, acting like a magnet to dirt, and provides a rich source of minerals for the skin. It also absorbs excess oil and helps to shrink open pores. Fuller's earth is one of the most popular types of clay used in face packs because of its deep-cleansing properties. Combined with jasmine, lavender, and oil of rose, it can be applied not only to the face but also the whole body to tighten the skin. Powdered white clay has strongly astringent qualities that help to firm up the skin and boost blood and lymph circulation.

Green clay is one of the most successful agents for restoring the bloom of youth to jaded skin. Used regularly, it helps to limit the spread of wrinkles by stimulating the muscles of the face and aiding the flow of blood and lymph. Another remarkable property of green clay is that it reduces the amount of sebum in oily skin and yet enriches normal skin. But if you have dry skin you should take care when using clay. It can be useful in removing toxins and dead cells but always add a hydrating substance to the mix such as olive oil, herbs or essential oils. Remove the mask as soon as you feel your skin beginning to pull.

It's easy to spend a small fortune on shop-bought masks but you can buy the basic ingredients at a fraction of the price to make your own cheap and healthy alternatives. You can find powdered clay in most health food and herb stores. To make your own mask more effective, select ingredients to suit your skin type. For example:

cucumber mask

This is for normal to oily skin.

INGREDIENTS:

4 tsp green clay
2 in (5 cm) piece of cucumber
2 tsp brewer's yeast

METHOD:

Put all the ingredients in a blender and mix until they form a smooth paste. If the mixture is too watery just add a little more clay. Apply to the face and leave on for 15–20 minutes. Wash off with warm water.

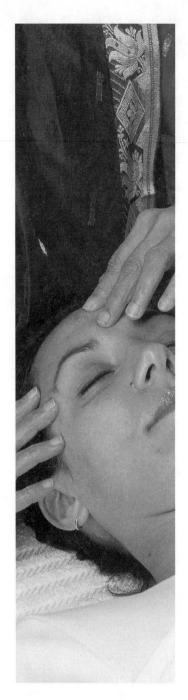

aloe vera mask

This is for normal to dry skin.

INGREDIENTS:

6 tsp clay
2 tsp aloe vera juice
1 egg white or spring water if you prefer
1 tsp honey

METHOD:

Mix all the ingredients together in a bowl to a moist but firm consistency. Apply to the face and leave for 10–20 minutes. Rinse off with warm water.

witch hazel mask

This is for combination or oily skin.

INGREDIENTS:

2 tsp Fuller's earth
2 tsp witch hazel
1 egg white, lightly beaten

METHOD:

Mix the Fuller's earth and witch hazel in a bowl to form a smooth paste and then add the egg white. Mix thoroughly and apply to the nose, chin, and forehead with a make-up brush. Leave for 5–10 minutes and rinse off.

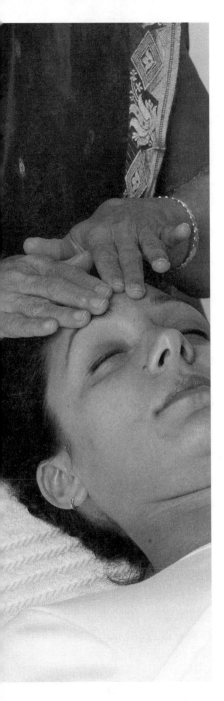

honey mask

This is for mature skin.

INGREDIENTS:

6 tsp clay
3 tsp honey
2 tsp aloe vera juice or spring water
A few drops of vitamin E and A
A few drops of evening primrose oil or borage oil

METHOD:

Mix all the ingredients in a bowl and apply to the face for about 15 minutes or until you feel the mask beginning to pull. Rinse off with warm water.

yogurt and jojoba mask

This is for blemished skin.

INGREDIENTS:

6 tsp clay
2 tsp jojoba oil
1 tsp yogurt

METHOD:

Mix all the ingredients in a bowl, apply to the face, leave for 20 minutes, and rinse off with warm water.

parsley and oil mask

This mask is for a mature neck.

INGREDIENTS:

2 tbsp fresh parsley

2 tbsp clay

1 tbsp olive oil

1 tbsp wheatgerm oil

2 tbsp witch hazel

METHOD:

Chop the parsley and put in a bowl with the clay. Stir in the olive oil and wheatgerm oil. Add the witch hazel and mix. Apply immediately. Leave on the face for about 30 minutes and then rinse off with warm water.

face packs

Face packs are a gentler version of face masks. They work in a similar manner by improving circulation and cleansing and tightening the skin. But they are more porous than masks and allow the skin to breathe, so they can be left on much longer. The following recipes use fruit and vegetables as their base in order to provide the vitamins and enzymes to rejuvenate, tone, balance, and cleanse the skin.

strawberry face pack

This is for all skin types.

METHOD:

Crush a few strawberries and apply straight to the face. Leave on for about 15 minutes and rinse off with warm water or rosewater. This mask has great revitalizing and toning properties but if you want an even stronger effect add 1 stiffly beaten egg white and 1 tablespoon rosewater to the mixture.

honey and banana face pack

This is for lacklustre and dehydrated skins.

INGREDIENTS:

1 small ripe banana
1 oz (25 g) finely ground oatmeal
1 tsp runny honey

METHOD:

Put the flesh of the banana into a bowl and mash to a smooth paste. Stir in the oatmeal and honey. Apply to the face and neck and leave for 15–20 minutes. Remove with damp cotton wool.

apricot face pack

This is for normal to dry skin.

METHOD:

Peel two fresh apricots and remove the stones. Put the flesh into a bowl and mash with a fork or use a food processor for a few seconds. Apply this straight to the face and leave for at least 30 minutes. Rinse off with cotton wool balls dipped in warm water or rosewater.

avocado face pack

This recipe can be varied to suit dry, combination, and mature skin. The basic recipe is for dry skin.

METHOD:

Put the flesh of a ripe avocado in a bowl and mash with a fork or use a food processor for a few seconds. Apply to the skin and leave for about 30 minutes. Rinse off with cotton wool balls dipped in warm water or rosewater.

This recipe includes egg yolk for combination skin.

METHOD:
Put the flesh of a ripe avocado in a bowl and mash with a fork or use a food processor for a few seconds. Add 1 beaten egg yolk and mix. Apply to the skin and leave on for about 30 minutes. Rinse off with cotton wool balls dipped in warm water or rosewater.

This recipe includes honey for aging skin.

METHOD:
Put the flesh of a ripe avocado in a bowl and mash with a fork or use a food processor for a few seconds. Add 1 tablespoon of honey and 1 beaten egg yolk and mix. Apply to the skin and leave on for about 30 minutes. Rinse off with cotton wool balls dipped in warm water or rosewater.

grape lotion

This lotion can be used daily to aid dry, aging or damaged skin.

METHOD:
Crush enough grapes with a fork to yield about 2 tablespoons of juice. Apply the juice to the face with cotton wool balls or a make-up brush. Leave on for about 20 minutes and wash off with rosewater.

apple tingler

This is for oily skin.

METHOD:
Grate the skin of one apple. Apply to the face and leave on for 30 minutes. Wash off with warm water. This leaves the skin feeling tingly and fresh.

orange astringent

This is for oily skin.

METHOD:
Peel an orange and boil the segments in water for 15 minutes. Leave to cool, then strain off the pulp and discard. Apply the remaining liquid to the face and leave for 30 minutes. Wash off with warm water. The liquid works wonders at removing the last traces of dirt, closing pores, and leaving the skin soft and smooth.

lemon astringent

Lemon works wonders on oily skin.

METHOD:
Add 1 teaspoon of freshly squeezed lemon juice to one stiffly beaten egg white. Apply to the skin and rinse off after about 10 minutes with warm water or rosewater.

glycerine and banana

This is for dry skin.

METHOD:
Peel a banana and mash in a bowl. Add 1 tablespoon of rosewater and two drops of glycerine. Mix well. Before putting on your make-up in the morning, apply the mixture to your face and leave on for 30 minutes. Wash off with warm water. Your skin will feel wonderfully supple for hours.

blackcurrant and yogurt

This is for normal and dry skin.

METHOD:
Place 3 tablespoons of blackcurrants in a bowl and crush with a fork. Add 2 tablespoons of live yogurt. Apply to the skin and leave on for at least 15 minutes. Rinse off with warm water or rosewater.

buying skincare products

If you don't have time to make your own beauty products or prefer to buy from a shop, you need to know what you're spending your money on. You can pay anything for a cleanser or moisturizer, but is it worth it? In a French study of anti-aging products, a budget vitamin E anti-wrinkle cream came out top for effectiveness, despite its bargain basement price. So, before you buy, always compare prices. Economical products may not come in fancy wrapping but they can have just as many useful properties as their more expensive counterparts.

The best guide to choosing the right product is how it feels on the skin. A moisturizer should be absorbed easily and not leave a greasy film behind. It's a good idea to choose one that gives a longer-lasting effect, and is fragrance- and color-free, as additives may irritate the skin.

Cleansers are available in a bewildering range including creams, lotions, rinse-off gels, and soap-free bars. You can also buy cleansers and toners combined, which saves time and money. Soap and water cleanses off water-soluble dirt, but its alkaline nature can upset the skin's natural pH (acid/alkaline) balance, leaving it dry and tight. Also, it is less effective at dissolving oil-based make-up or removing excess sebum from the skin.

A sign of a good cleanser is that it should easily remove all impurities, such as oil, grime, make-up, and loose skin cells. Also, it should not leave a residue that can clog pores and cause spots. In general, wash-off cleansers are best suited to oilier skin types and cream-based ones to drier skins. If you have sensitive skin, avoid products containing soap, fragrance, and color.

Night creams contain more active ingredients than daily moisturizers as the skin is supposedly more receptive and cell renewal more active when we're at rest. They also tend to be richer (or thicker) and this is more acceptable for night-time use. If you have oily or combination skin, your normal daytime moisturizer will probably do just as well, although night creams do have a higher concentration of herbal and vitamin extracts.

When buying skincare products, always study the list of ingredients so you know what the item is intended to do. The following are some of the most commonly used ingredients. They can be highly effective and rarely cause adverse reactions. However, if any product causes inflammation, a rash or any other unpleasant side-effect, stop using it immediately and, if necessary, seek medical advice.

- ❧ *Alpha hydroxy acids (AHAs): These are derived from natural substances such as milk, papaya, and apples. AHAs aid exfoliation and cell renewal by dissolving the natural adhesive that holds dead cells on to the surface of the skin. They also help diminish fine lines and brighten the complexion. However, recent research has shown that they may have a damaging effect and actually hasten skin aging. Further research is being carried out to try to resolve this issue.*
- ❧ *Antioxidants: These are substances such as beta-carotene and the vitamins A, C, and E that protect the skin against free radicals which can be produced by the sun, pollution, or cigarette smoke, or occur naturally in the body. Some experts claim that antioxidants prevent wrinkles, too. Vitamin E can also help repair sunburnt or sun-damaged skin.*
- ❧ *Ascorbic Acid: This is the scientific name for vitamin C and has been found to aid skin healing, reduce fine lines, and increase skin plumpness by stimulating the production of collagen and elastin.*
- ❧ *Ceramides: These lipids (fats) are found between the top layers of skin cells and help to retain moisture. Products containing ceramides are best for dry, mature or sun-damaged skin.*

- **Co-enzyme Q10:** This is one of the most recent "miracle" ingredients to appear in skin creams. It is a highly potent antioxidant that also fights bacteria. Q10 is believed to help to reduce wrinkles and improve the skin's elasticity and firmness.

- **Collagen and elastin:** Fibers of these proteins make up the main structural components of the connective tissue, giving the skin strength and flexibility. They are added to products to rejuvenate or replace the skin's naturally occurring proteins.

- **Glycolic Acid:** Derived from sugar cane, glycolic acid is said to be the simplest and smallest AHA. It is mainly used in skincare products to treat acne scars and other blemishes.

- **Humectants:** These chemicals draw moisture out of the air and so they are invaluable in moisturizers and facial sprays for dry skin. Common humectants include glycerine, sorbitol, squalene, and urea.

- **Liposomes:** Developed to deliver medication to specific areas of the body, liposomes carry nourishment deeper into the upper skin layer to plump it up and help prevent fine lines.

- **Panthenol (pro-vitamin B5):** This is one of the B complex vitamins and has been used in skin and hair products for over a decade. It helps to plump up and condition the skin.

- **Retinol, tretinoin, or retinoic acid:** These are the scientific names for natural and synthetic vitamin A. Originally used to treat acne, they are also effective against lines, wrinkles, and sun-damaged skin and so have become key ingredients in many skincare products. Research has shown that they can speed up production of epidermal cells and collagen and elastin fibers, even-out discoloration, and improve skin texture. They must be used with care as they can increase the skin's sensitivity to the sun.

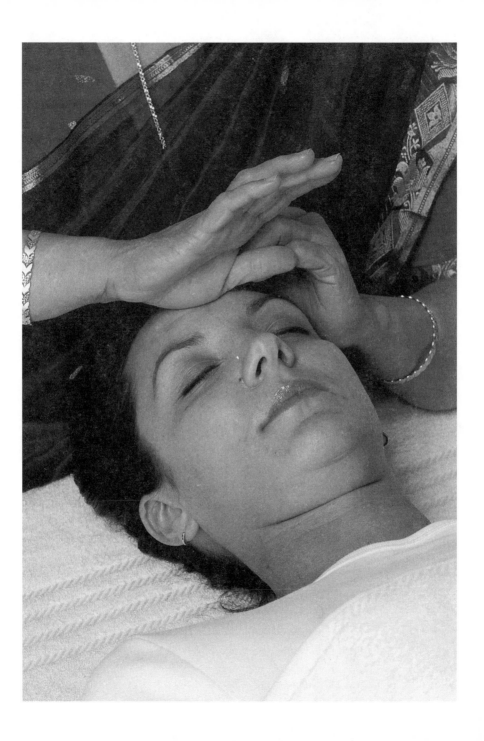

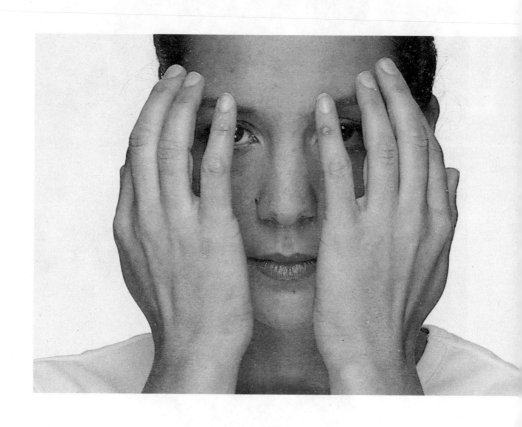

beauty from within

feeding the inner self

Followers of Ayurveda believe that beauty comes from within; that your "inner self" determines your outward appearance. So what you put into your body will have a huge impact on the way you look. The expression "you are what you eat" has become a cliché but that doesn't mean it's not as true today as it ever was.

Your diet determines how quickly your skin ages, and no moisturizing cream, no matter how expensive, can reverse the damage caused by years of poor eating habits. To function and develop properly, your skin cells need a constant supply of nutrients. In addition to following a regular skincare routine, the best way to improve the condition of the skin and to keep it looking younger for longer is to feed it a well-balanced diet. In this chapter we look at the importance of eating the right kinds of foods, to make sure you take in all the nutrients your body needs.

To keep your skin looking young and vibrant you should aim to increase your intake of fresh fruit and vegetables and unrefined or unprocessed food. It's also a good idea to drink a glass of fresh fruit or vegetable juice every day. You'll see and feel the difference in only a few days. Your body will contain more of the essential vitamins and minerals you need to stay healthy and you'll be well rewarded with good-looking skin. The quality of the food you put into your body shows itself on your skin. Highly processed foods usually lack fiber but contain high levels of saturated fats, dubious additives, and refined sugar that the body regards as toxic and tries to reject by producing spots. Your complexion also looks dull and lifeless.

Eating too much can age you, too, particularly if your diet contains highly processed foods and animal proteins. Consuming more than your body needs encourages a build-up of waste matter and increases the production of toxins within the system. Your aim should be to eat less, but more healthily. But be wary of following the latest "fad" diet or one that is too austere as this can lead to deficiencies in vital nutrients. This also shows up on your face.

vanity vitamins

We have already said that antioxidant vitamins in fruit and vegetables can work wonders when applied to the skin. But it is even more important to ensure that your diet contains plenty of these essential nutrients. Many people who lead hectic lives and so live on fast food and snacks now take supplements to ensure

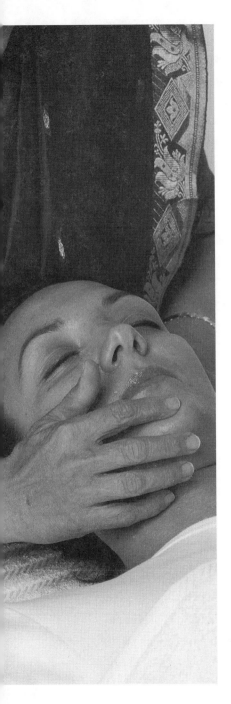

an adequate intake of vitamins and minerals.
But it is much better to obtain them from
natural food sources. Remember: fruit is the
original fast food – and the healthiest – and
raw vegetables make tasty and nutritious
snacks when you're in a hurry. Research
shows that smokers often eat a diet that is low
in antioxidant vitamins even though their
need for these nutrients is higher than that of
non-smokers.

the ACE nutrients

The most effective antioxidant vitamins are A,
C, and E. Ensuring your diet contains
adequate amounts of these protective nutrients
will bring many health benefits, and not just
to your skin.

❧ *A (retinol): This is necessary for healthy skin
and tissues and keeps the skin smooth and
supple. A deficiency may lead to dull, flaky
skin, premature wrinkles, skin disorders, and
lowered resistance to infection. Good food
sources include dairy products, liver, margarine,
and oily fish. But bear in mind that vitamin A
is stored in the body and an excess can be
harmful, especially to an unborn child.
Therefore pregnant women are advised to avoid
the richest sources of vitamin A, such as liver, or
supplements containing this nutrient, except on
their physician's advice. Vitamin A is made in
the body from carotenes, which are plant*

pigments found in bright-colored fruit and vegetables such as apricots, broccoli, carrots, oranges, peppers, and spinach. Pregnant women can safely eat as much as they like of these foods.

- ❊ **C (ascorbic acid):** *This is an important vitamin for healthy skin. As well as being an effective antioxidant, it is vital for the production of collagen, the main structural protein in the skin, and for tissue repair and renewal. Good food sources include blackcurrant, broccoli, Brussels sprouts, citrus fruit, green vegetables, potatoes, rosehip syrup, and tomatoes.*

- ❊ **E (tocopherols):** *Dry, flaking skin can be a tell-tale sign that your diet lacks vitamin E. This vitamin is regarded as the most important antioxidant for preventing free-radical damage to the skin and resisting premature aging. Some experts say that a diet rich in sources of vitamin E helps to repair sun-damaged skin. Vitamin E can be depleted by the hormone oestrogen, so if you are taking the pill or having hormone replacement therapy (HRT) you may have to increase your intake of this nutrient. Good food sources include brown rice, broccoli, cereals, eggs, green leafy vegetables, unrefined vegetable oils, such as sunflower and safflower, and wholegrains, particularly wheatgerm.*

more skin-boosters

A healthy diet should contain adequate amounts of all the nutrients, but there are certain vitamins, in addition to those already mentioned, that are particularly useful for healthy skin but that may be lacking in some diets.

- ❊ **B2 (riboflavin):** *This vitamin is essential for the repair and maintenance of the tissues. If your diet is deficient in B2, your tissues will regenerate more slowly, which eventually shows up as dry, wrinkled patches of skin, cracked lips, and even hair loss. Good food sources include breakfast cereals, dairy foods, fish, mushrooms, shellfish, and wheatgerm.*

- ❊ **B3 (niacin):** *This is another vitamin that is important for the maintenance of healthy skin. If it is deficient in the diet the skin may become rough and flaky. Good food sources include asparagus, chicken, dairy foods, green leafy vegetables, liver, nuts, oily fish, peas, potatoes, and red meats.*

- ❀ **B5 (pantothenic acid):** *This vitamin has anti-aging properties, especially when combined with antioxidants. Good food sources include egg yolk, liver, nuts, wheatgerm, wheat bran, and yeast extract.*

- ❀ **B6 (pyridoxine):** *Best known as the anti-stress vitamin, B6 is important for cell oxidation and tissue repair and growth. It is also thought to improve the symptoms of pre-menstrual syndrome (PMS). Low levels can exacerbate both dry and oily skin conditions, and lead to dandruff, rashes, and other skin disorders. This is another vitamin that is depleted by oestrogen, so consider increasing your intake of B6 if you take the pill or are having HRT. Good food sources include avocado, bananas, breakfast cereals, broccoli, cabbage, cauliflower, dried beans, nuts, oily fish, pork, sesame seeds, turkey, and wheatgerm, including wholewheat bread.*

- ❀ **Choline:** *One of the B vitamins, this nutrient plays a part in the repair and renewal of skin cells, so keeping the skin looking young. Good food sources include eggs, nuts, pulses, citrus fruits, and leafy vegetables.*

- ❀ **H (biotin):** *This vitamin helps to make energy available from food, especially for the removal of the waste products of protein and the synthesis of fats. Eating foods rich in this nutrient can improve skin conditions such as dermatitis. Good food sources include egg yolk, kidney, liver, mushrooms, nuts, oats, soya, and wheatgerm.*

minerals for healthy skin

Some minerals and trace elements are particularly important for the well-being of the skin. But many of the following may be deficient in some diets, especially if the food you eat is grown in impoverished soil.

- ❀ **Copper:** *This mineral is important for the manufacture of connective tissue and the skin pigment melanin. It is contained in collagen and elastin and helps ensure smooth, clear skin. It is also part of the body's antioxidant enzyme superoxide dismutase and so helps to prevent premature aging. Good food sources include curry powder, liver, seafood, and wholegrains.*

- ❀ **Iodine:** *This is a vital constituent of thyroid hormones, which regulate the body's metabolism and control growth. A deficiency of this mineral can have many dire effects on the body, including extreme fatigue, as well as causing course, flaky, dry skin and* hair. Many people lack an adequate intake of this mineral. Good food sources include iodized table salt, seafood such as shellfish, and seaweed (see "kelp" on following page.)

- ❀ **Magnesium:** *This mineral helps to build up the skin's connective tissue. It also plays a role in the formation of glycoproteins, a combination of glucose and protein molecules, which are a major component of cells. Good food sources include avocado, green leafy vegetables, nuts, pineapples, seeds, soya, and wholewheat bread.*

- ❀ **Selenium:** *This mineral is vital for strong, healthy, and supple tissues and works with vitamin E to combat free-radical damage. It may be lacking in foods such as cereals that are grown in selenium-deficient soil. Good food sources include brazil nuts, fish, meat, seafood, seaweed, and wholegrains.*

- ❀ **Silicon:** *This is present in minute quantities in connective tissue and helps keep the skin supple, elastic, strong, and healthy. The best sources are organically grown produce, particularly vegetables.*

- ❀ **Sulphur:** *This element is a constituent of vitamin B1 and certain amino acids, the building blocks from which proteins are made. It is needed for the manufacture of collagen, the main structural protein of the dermis, and keratin, the main component of the epidermis and hair. It is found in horseradish, kidney beans, peas, and shellfish.*

- ❀ **Zinc:** *This plays a part in numerous cellular reactions in tissues throughout the body. It promotes skin repair, strengthens elastin and collagen fibers, and protects against skin problems such as acne, helping to maintain a clear and healthy complexion. It is also an antioxidant. Good food sources include beans, dairy foods, eggs, hard cheese, lean meat, nuts, pumpkin seeds, shellfish, sunflower seeds, wholewheat bread, and yogurt.*

Alternative skin enhancers

Some plants that do not usually form a part of the normal diet are very rich in nutrients or have other important skin-enhancing properties.

❀ Alfalfa: The sprouted seeds of this plant provide a wealth of nutrients that keep the skin healthy. It is a good source of chlorophyll, which aids wound repair; important amino acids; vitamins, especially B vitamins; minerals such as calcium; and several enzymes that aid digestion. To gain the optimum benefits be sure to eat the seeds after germination.

❀ Echinacea: This is a herbal extract taken from a flower that grows in North America and is traditionally used to fight infection. It works by stimulating white blood cells, increasing their activity and number. As a skincare aid, it stimulates the regeneration of connective tissue and epidermal cells and accelerates wound healing.

❀ Kelp: This is a type of seaweed rich in iodine, a mineral that is often deficient in foods grown in upland areas where it is easily washed out of the soil. Iodine and other nutrients found in kelp aid the removal of toxins from the body, so helping to maintain a clear complexion.

fats – good guys and bad guys

Fats in the diet provide a concentrated form of energy and also give food a pleasant and satisfying taste. But not all fats are the same – there are "bad guys" and "good guys." The bad guys are saturated fats such as butter, lard, cheese, whole milk, cream, and fatty cuts of meat. Although dairy products and meat are important sources of many vitamins and minerals, where possible choose low-fat versions. Generally in the West we eat far too many foods that are high in saturated fats, leading to clogged arteries and heart disease. Fats are transported in the body via the lymphatic system so an excess intake in the diet can restrict the flow of lymph and reduce its ability to fight disease and remove toxins from the body, leaving your skin looking dull and unhealthy. Saturated fats also increase the risk of clogged pores in people with oily skin, resulting in a spotty complexion. You should also avoid fried or barbecued food as these destroy antioxidants in the body.

The good guys are the unsaturated fats. These come in two main forms: monounsaturated, found in avocado, olive oil, and sesame oil, and polyunsaturated, found in soya beans, oily fish, nuts, seeds, and the oils made from them. Unsaturated fats are a rich source of vitamins such as A, D, E, and K and special nutrients called essential fatty acids (EFAs). As the name suggests, essential fatty acids are vital for health but they cannot be manufactured by the body, so they must be obtained from the diet.

There are two essential fatty acids that are particularly important for the skin. These are omega-6 linoleic acid and omega-3 alpha-linolenic acid. They are important components of cellular membranes and are also needed for the synthesis of signalling molecules, such as the prostaglandins. EFAs are converted by the body into other forms. Linoleic acid is converted into gamma-linoleic acid (GLA) which is particularly important for healthy skin. GLA helps to strengthen the skin, increases the moisture content of cells, and speeds up the rejuvenation process. It also aids the production of strong collagen and elastin fibers in the dermis, helping to prevent wrinkles and sagging. Supplements such as evening primrose oil ensure that you have enough GLA in your body.

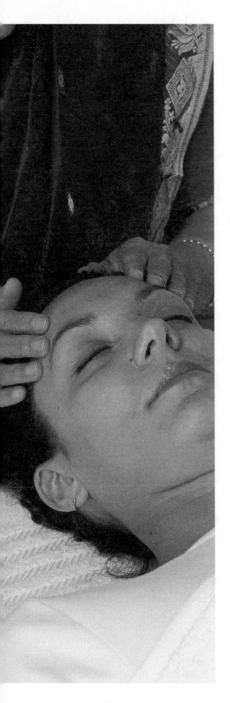

You can increase your intake of unsaturated fats by adding one tablespoon of unrefined, uncooked vegetable oil, such as extra virgin olive oil, to salad dressing or sauces poured over pasta or boiled potatoes. Tinned oily fish such as sardines, mackerel, and salmon are also very rich in EFAs.

The effect of upping your intake of EFAs can take 4–6 weeks to show on your skin but you'll notice the difference – especially after a bath, or when you've spent some time outdoors on a windy day, as your skin will feel less tight and will look softer. EFAs can also delay or prevent the appearance of wrinkles. It is important to reduce your intake of saturated and processed fats as these cancel out the effects of EFAs in your body.

the wonder of water

The body is made up mostly of water but you are constantly losing this vital fluid in the breath, via perspiration, and when you urinate. An adequate supply of water is essential to purify the system, help vital organs function well, and retain adequate moisture levels in skin cells. Dehydration can cause us to feel sluggish, lethargic, and easily fatigued. The skin dries out more quickly and becomes more prone to premature wrinkling. Ideally you should drink 50–70 fl oz/1.5–2 liters every day. This not only helps to replace the fluid you've lost but also helps the kidneys to flush out toxins from the system. Once you start to increase your daily water intake you'll notice the difference in a week. Your skin will be clearer and any dark circles around your eyes, which indicate that your kidneys are having a hard time dealing with the toxins in your body, will soon disappear.

You should filter your tap water or buy low-sodium-content mineral water as too much sodium (a constituent of salt) can dehydrate you. In addition, drink a glass or two of freshly squeezed fruit or vegetable juice every day. Raw fruit juices are packed full of nutrients including enzymes, which are easily destroyed by heat and light. Herbal teas are a healthy alternative to caffeinated teas and coffee, which tend to increase fluid loss from the body leading to dehydration.

dietary demons

Apart from saturated fats, there are other "demons in the diet" that can have adverse effects on the skin. In particular, many people in the West consume far too much alcohol, salt, and refined sugar for the good of their skin – and their general health. These needn't be eliminated from the diet, indeed salt is vital, but you should limit your intake.

alcohol

A moderate amount of alcohol per day, such as a glass of red wine, is thought to be good for you as it is said to have a protective effect on the heart and cardiovascular system. But in excess, alcohol is bad news for the skin. It dehydrates you by increasing the amount you sweat and urinate, draining the tissues of vital moisture, and accelerating skin aging. Alcohol is high in calories and also encourages the consumption of snacks and junk foods that are loaded with fats, sugar, and salt but low in essential nutrients.

salt

The typical Western diet contains too much salt. We add it to cooking, to the food on our plate, and it is present in most processed foods. Even some sweet foods, such as biscuits, contain salt. But too much salt overloads the kidneys, impairing their ability to filter impurities from the blood and increasing fluid retention. This causes bags under the eyes and cellulite.

sugar

The West is a big consumer of sugar. Refined table sugar, or sucrose, and simple sugars such as glucose, maltose, and dextrose are found in many processed foods. For example, tomato ketchup is 15 percent sugar. Eating too much sugar has been linked to skin conditions such as acne, poor skin quality, and lowered immunity. Over-consumption can affect glucose regulation systems, leading to a problem called protein glycation (see page 30) that is thought to be a principal cause of age-related skin damage. Your skin will thank you if you can wean yourself off sweet foods.

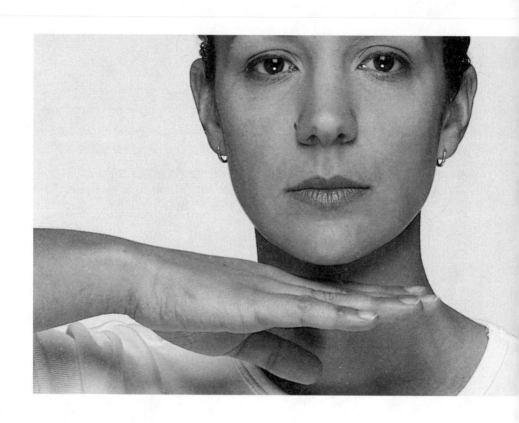

managing your life

stress, sleeplessness, smoking, and sun

Diet is not the only aspect of your lifestyle that can damage your skin. Stress, lack of sleep, cigarette smoking, and sunbathing can all have an adverse effect on the way you look. If you are under stress you may not be sleeping properly. Your appetite can be affected, so you don't eat properly.

You may increase your alcohol intake and start smoking. A combination of factors like these is a common cause of premature skin aging.

stress

Stress is invariably regarded as the villain of the piece and the root cause of everything bad in our lives. But it's important to remember that stress, when managed well, can be a force for good, helping us to become stronger and wiser. When you come through a stressful situation you may find that the world seems a different place and your priorities have changed. You can often learn valuable lessons from a stressful experience and may even look forward to similar challenges so you can put what you have learned into practice.

However, chronic unresolved stress is another matter and must be dealt with, or it can lead to severe illness. Stress raises the levels of the "fight or flight" hormones – cortisol, adrenaline, and noradrenaline – in the body. These hormones prepare the body for physical exertion by, for example, releasing glucose and fatty acids into the bloodstream and increasing the heart and breathing rate. For your ancestors, living at a time when stressful situations were more straightforward – such as fighting a band of marauding tribesmen or fleeing from a wild animal – stress was vital for survival. Once the crisis was over, the stress hormones dispersed naturally. Today, the most common causes of stress are not resolved so easily. They can include work or financial worries, relationship problems, bereavement, or a serious illness in the family. If the stressful situation can't be resolved, the stress hormones continue to circulate in the bloodstream, keeping the body in a constant state of high alert.

effects of stress

Chronic stress has numerous adverse effects on the body, many of which can influence the way you look. It can lead to disturbed sleep and insomnia, for example, which inhibits the repair and renewal of the skin. The anxiety and tension you feel will be reflected in your face, which remains in a perpetual frown. The lack of facial muscle movement causes fluid and toxins to accumulate in the tissues, leaving you looking pale and puffy. Your face starts to look drawn with dull eyes and a dull complexion.

The stress hormone cortisol also switches off the immune system, leaving you vulnerable to a wide range of illnesses, including skin infections and spots. The level of glucose and fatty acids in the bloodstream remains constantly high, as they are not being burned up by the extreme physical exertion your body is geared up for. This accelerates skin damage caused by protein glycation (see page 30) and increases the amount of fat that is deposited in the blood vessels, leading to circulation problems.

tackling stress

Work problems are among the most common causes of stress and can affect an office junior just as much as a managing director. Work stress can be a consequence of working in a job that is not really suited to your skills or temperament, or stretches you too much – or not enough. You may not get on with colleagues or may feel that your boss doesn't appreciate you. Two out of three consultations with physicians concern stress-related illness, so the sooner you recognize a problem, the earlier it can be resolved.

self-help for stress

There are short-term and long-term measures you can use to help you manage stress. Short-term measures only offer temporary relief, however, so don't delay too long before dealing with the underlying cause.

- *Take five: Whenever you feel seriously stressed you should take a short break and try to relax. Just 2–3 minutes away from the workplace can help. Read a book, or take a stroll in the open air – it's amazing the difference a walk can make. Anything that takes your mind off work for a few minutes can reduce stress levels.*
- *Have a chat: Talk to someone about the way you're feeling and the underlying concerns that are contributing to your stress. You can chat to friends, colleagues or partners. They may offer useful advice, but even if they have no practical suggestions, talking over your worries can help put them in perspective.*

Physical signs of stress

Stress affects people in different ways – indeed some people are unaware that they're under stress. The following are some of the most common physical symptoms and signs of stress. They act as a warning, suggesting that stress is becoming a serious problem. The more signs you are experiencing, the more stress you are under.

High blood pressure/palpitations

Hyperventilation

Excess sweating

Poor skin condition

Stiff, aching, tense muscles

Disturbed sleep pattern

Headaches

Anxiety

Depression

Poor hair condition

Loss of appetite

Tiredness

Low sex drive

Emotional signs of stress

Some behaviour patterns can indicate stress. However, as with physical symptoms, emotional responses can differ between individuals. One person may be overwhelmed and constantly tearful, while another may become argumentative, aggressive or petulant. It is important to recognize a problem behaviour pattern and confront the issues that may be causing it. Ask yourself whether any of the following symptoms apply to you.

Irritability
Loss of sense of humor
Low self-esteem
Feelings of helplessness
Loneliness
Difficulty concentrating
Confusion
Comfort eating
Forgetfulness
Nightmares
Panic attacks
Relationship problems
Starting or increasing smoking
Eating disorders, such as skipping meals and/or bingeing
Gambling/taking needless risks
Alcohol binges or dependence

- 🌸 **Think caffeine-free:** *Avoid caffeinated coffee or tea at times of stress. These are stimulants and can exacerbate feelings of anxiety and tension. A better option is to drink herbal tea or mineral water.*
- 🌸 **Have a snack:** *Many people find that a carbohydrate snack makes them feel better when under stress. The brain produces a chemical, serotonin, which induces happy, feel-good emotions. Serotonin is made from an amino acid called tryptophan, found in foods such as almonds, meat, peanuts, sesame seeds, tahini (sesame seed paste), and tofu. Tryptophan is absorbed into the brain more efficiently if there is plenty of carbohydrate present. However, always choose low-fat, low sugar snacks such as unbuttered toasted bread, raw vegetables and fruit, otherwise snacking can lead to further problems, such as unwanted weight gain and spots.*
- 🌸 **Happy thoughts:** *Just thinking about a funny situation or something or someone who amuses you can release tension and lift your mood. A laugh and a joke with friends or colleagues is best, or read a humorous book or magazine, or watch a comedy film or video.*

prioritize and delegate

Remember, you're only human and can't be expected to do everything. If you are getting bogged down with work or find you have taken on too many tasks you'll need to prioritize and, where necessary, delegate. Make a list of the tasks you can realistically complete the following day. You'll feel an immense sense of satisfaction as you tick off each task as it's completed. Less important tasks can be left to another time, or ask someone else to help you. If you're not getting on well with a colleague or family member, perhaps it's because they feel undervalued. Asking for help is not a sign of failure but shows you trust others to do a good job.

office exercises

One sign of stress is muscular tension, especially in the neck, shoulders, and back. Taking a break from work to play sport or spend an hour in the gym is a good way to deal with this problem, but may not be a realistic option on a busy day. However, if you work in an office you'll find that the following simple exercises are great for correcting your posture, relieving tension, and helping you to relax. They'll give your mind a workout too, improving your concentration and mental well-being, so you work more effectively. Make the workout part of your daily routine. You can do some of the exercises when you have a few minutes to yourself, either at lunch or when you're feeling bogged down and unable to cope. You'll notice a change in your mood after just a few days. The workout, which can be done at your desk, only takes about 10 minutes, so it can be fitted in to the most hectic work schedule.

preparation

Prepare by sitting straight on a chair with your shoulders back, hands on your lap, and both feet on the ground. Repeat all the exercises three times. Do not strain. Breathe in as you perform the action and breathe out as you return to the starting position.

neck stretch

This releases neck tension and improves mobility and suppleness.

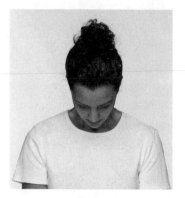

Sit looking straight ahead and gently bring your head towards your chest as far as it will go. Hold for three seconds and return to the starting position. Repeat.

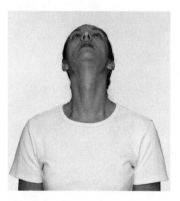

Gently take your head back as far as you can. Hold for three seconds and then release. Repeat.

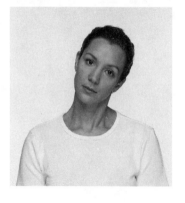

Lower your head towards your left shoulder, keeping your right shoulder down. Hold for five seconds and release. Repeat. Now repeat on the right side.

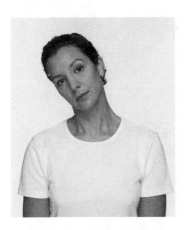

Now repeat on the other side.

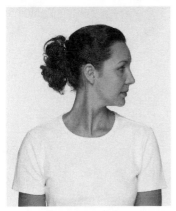

Turn your head to look over your left shoulder as far as possible without moving your body. Hold for three seconds then release.

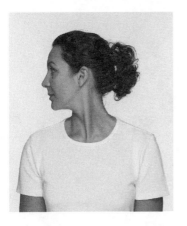

Repeat on the right side.

shoulder lift

This exercise releases muscular tension in the shoulders and increases mobility, as well as improving posture.

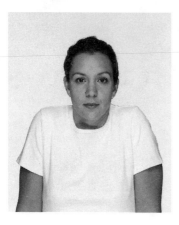

Take a deep breath and lift both shoulders as high as you can. Hold for three seconds then breathe out as you lower. Repeat.

arm stretch

This exercise releases tension in the upper arms and shoulders and improves flexibility and mobility.

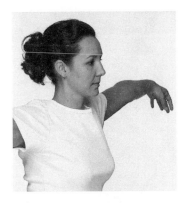

Breathe in as you stretch your arms out to the side. Then shake your wrists and fingers.

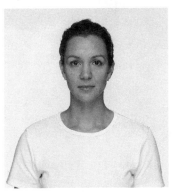

Breathe out as you let your arms fall by your sides. Repeat.

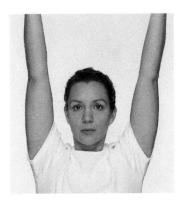

Breathe in as you raise your arms to the ceiling. Breathe out as you lower your arms to your sides.

eye rest

This is an excellent exercise for relieving eye strain and tension headaches.

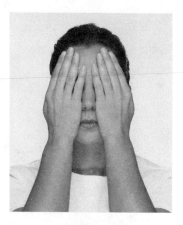

Rest your elbows on the desk and cover your eyes with your hands. Don't hunch your shoulders up – keep them down and relaxed.

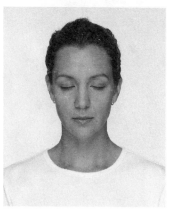

Keeping your eyes and mouth closed, take three slow, deep breaths, breathing in and out only through your nose. Then rest. Repeat.

mental relaxation exercise

Once you have practiced the physical exercises, combine them with the following mental relaxation exercise to improve your mental well-being. This exercise can calm you, improve your concentration, and allow you to become more focused. You'll feel your mind clear of stress and tension.

Sit comfortably but straight with your shoulders back and down and your feet on the floor. Keeping your head level, close your eyes, and concentrate on your breathing. Breathe slowly and rhythmically through your nose. Imagine you are in a peaceful place surrounded by beautiful scenery. It could be a favorite weekend retreat or vacation venue, such as a secluded beach or a tranquil woodland glade in the countryside, or somewhere that exists only in your imagination. Relax and think about the colors and smells and enjoy the soothing environment. You'll soon feel calm and relaxed. Stay in this position for 5–10 minutes. When you're ready, open your eyes and stretch your arms, first at shoulder level and then above your head.

long-term solutions

The following measures can help provide a more permanent solution to chronic stress. But you will also need to tackle any underlying issues.

take exercise

As the job of the stress hormones is to get your body ready for physical effort, regular exercise can act as a valuable safety valve, "burning off" the glucose and fatty acids circulating round your body and releasing tension. Exercise also increases production of endorphins, "feel-good" chemicals that occur naturally in the body. These chemicals act like morphine (the name "endorphins" is short for "endogenous [naturally occurring] morphines") to ease physical and emotional pain and lighten mood.

In today's high-powered, highly competitive work environment you may put exercise to the bottom of your priority list. What's more, when feeling stressed you may not have much energy and enthusiasm for working out. However, it's well worth making the effort. Regular exercise not only helps control your stress levels, it also improves your general health. If you focus on the benefits that come with a regular exercise regime it can help you to maintain your resolve whenever your enthusiasm starts to flag. Why not encourage your partner, or a friend or colleague to exercise with you so you can provide mutual support.

If the gym doesn't appeal, consider other options like swimming, cycling or playing an energetic sport. A brisk walk for 30 minutes every day – in your lunch break, for example – can really give you a lift. Your mental state will be improved, you'll feel more energetic, and you'll have more enthusiasm for life. And, as if that wasn't enough, after a couple of months your body will seem more trim and lithe, your skin will look great, and you'll sleep more soundly, too!

balance work and play

How much of your personal time do you spend thinking about work? It is hard to switch off when you are stressed. But if you add up the minutes you spend in a typical week fretting over work problems you'll find it adds up to hours of wasted time that are better spent in recreational pursuits. Look at how you fill your day and think how you can change the balance. You may think you don't have time to see old friends but an evening out could be just what you need to help you wind down and view your worries in a new light. You need work and play to keep your life balanced and healthy.

it's good to listen

Make time to listen - not just to other people but to yourself as well. This can be hard, especially when your mind is cluttered with other matters. When talking to someone else, clear your head of all other thoughts and concentrate on their words. Spend a few seconds thinking about what they have said before you respond. It's perhaps even more important – and harder – to listen to yourself. Think about how you are feeling and what is causing you to feel that way. Make notes if necessary and give each worry a number between one and ten according to how much an issue troubles you. This helps to identify the problems that are causing most stress.

let stress work for you

Use stress to maximize your potential rather than letting it control you. You can never avoid all stress – and nor should you. Stress adds zest to life: it provides life's challenges, and the satisfaction of achievement when you conquer them. Managed well, stress helps you focus on a problem, meet a deadline, learn from mistakes, and tackle future problems more effectively.

tackling sleep problems

Sleep is vital for your mental and physical well-being. During sleep your body undertakes the vital tasks of mental and physical repair and renewal. After a good night's sleep you feel relaxed, refreshed, and energetic, and this shows in your face. It's no coincidence that many models insist on an early night before an important photographic shoot. In India, sleep is called "the wet nurse of the world" because of its regenerating, nourishing, and nurturing effects. A good night's sleep is essential for healthy living and good skin – it's not called "beauty sleep" for nothing. Your body needs time to rest and recuperate; while you sleep your skin develops new cells and healing takes place.

There are two types of sleep: dream sleep, which is also known as rapid eye movement sleep, because the eyes dart around in their sockets, and sound sleep, which is also called slow-wave sleep, because the brain produces slow waves of electrical activity. During dream sleep your mind is as active as if you were awake, whereas during sound sleep your brain shows much less activity. It is thought that mind and body are repaired, renewed, and replenished during slow-wave sleep. We alternate between both types of sleep during the night.

Dreams may occur in either phase, but are more likely to be remembered and to wake you during dream sleep. If you've been having vivid or emotion-charged dreams throughout the night you may get up after a long period of sleep still feeling very tired.

People vary in the amount of sleep they need. As you get older, your sleep pattern changes. You tend to need less sleep, and may take longer to get to sleep or wake up more often during the night. Lack of sleep for whatever reason – be it pleasure- or stress-related – can take its toll on your face and leave you looking and feeling drained. Studies show that insomnia and disturbed sleep are growing problems. Managing stress can help, but there are other measures that you can try if you are having difficulty getting to sleep, or find that you keep waking up in the night, or wake up too early in the morning. If you try the steps outlined below and find that your sleep pattern has still not improved, seek your physician's advice.

set your sleep pattern

The most important step is to keep to a fixed sleep routine. Your body clock works to a cyclic pattern of roughly 24 hours, known as the circadian rhythm. It is important to establish a fixed sleep pattern to keep your body clock set to the right time. When you have irregular sleeping and waking times your body clock is constantly being altered and you become alert or sleepy at all the wrong times. You should get into the habit of going to bed at the same time each night and arising at the same time each morning – even if you've had a restless night.

If you can't get to sleep after 10–15 minutes, don't just lie there – get out of bed until you feel sleepy. Try reading a relaxing (or boring!) book, or write a few letters. You must learn to associate bed with calm and relaxation, not anxiety and restlessness. Even if it takes an hour or more before you start to feel sleepy, get up at your normal time in the morning. Don't be tempted to have a lie-in to make up for lost sleep, even at the weekend, and try to avoid daytime naps, or you'll disrupt your sleep pattern and the problem will continue. If you must take a nap, have it in the afternoon and limit it to 15 minutes (set an alarm clock if necessary).

food for sleep

What you eat before you go to bed – and when – can affect the quality of your sleep. You should eat at least two hours before bedtime and try to avoid heavy meals in the evening. It is healthier to make lunch your main meal of the day. Some vitamins, minerals, and other supplements have a stimulant effect on the body, so take them in the morning rather than the evening unless there are specific instructions to do otherwise.

There is a close link between sleep and foods such as pasta, potatoes, and bread that are rich in complex carbohydrates. Such foods act like a natural sleeping pill, relaxing mind and body and preparing it for sleep. They stimulate the production of chemicals that not only make you feel sleepy but also stop you fidgeting in your sleep. If you find that a bowl of spaghetti at lunch slows you down, base your midday meal on a protein-rich diet, and save the complex carbohydrates for the evening.

Avoid eating too much refined sugar in the evening. Whether in the form of a malted bedtime drink, squash, chocolate, cookies or a sweet dessert, sugar acts as a stimulant, providing a sudden rush of energy that can keep you awake. Children's bodies are particularly sensitive to the rapid energy swings caused by excess sugar, but adults too can find that eating too much sugar leads to a disturbed night's sleep. If you like a dessert in the evening, choose one that includes fresh or dried fruit or wholewheat flour, which will slow down the rate at which the sugar enters your bloodstream. If you like a warm drink at bedtime, try herbal teas, such as camomile, rose petal and rose leaves, which promote restful sleep.

steps to good sleep

Here are some more simple steps you can try, to ensure restful and therapeutic sleep.

❀ **Check the temperature**. *Make sure the bedroom is neither too hot nor too cold, and ensure there is a little ventilation.*

❀ **Get a good bed**. *Invest in a comfortable bed, mattress, and pillow.*

❀ **Check your medicines**. *Certain medications such as cough mixtures and some anti-depressants can disrupt your sleep pattern. If you think this is the case talk to your physician, who may be able to change your medication.*

❀ **Avoid caffeine in the afternoon and evening**. *This includes colas, as well as tea and coffee. Even cocoa can act as a stimulant.*

❀ **Skip the night-cap**. *You may think alcohol helps you get a good night's sleep — unfortunately it doesn't. Alcohol is a stimulant and so can keep you awake or cause disturbed sleep that leaves you feeling drained in the morning. It will also dehydrate you, which is especially bad for the skin.*

❀ **Bathe away your worries**. *Just before going to bed, have a relaxing bath in your favorite aromatherapy oils. This will soothe away any nagging worries you have and allow you to sleep soundly. Put a few drops of lavender oil on a handkerchief and place it inside your pillow. The aroma of lavender is very soothing.*

❀ **Stop fretting**. *There is little you can do about a worrying situation while you're lying in bed so don't bottle it up. Talk it over with your partner, or chat to a friend or colleague the following day. Use the visualization technique (page 163) to clear your mind and help you to relax.*

❀ **Don't exercise too close to bedtime**. *You may find its effects are more stimulating than relaxing.*

smoking

Cigarette smoking is one of the main causes of skin aging and wrinkling. Women smokers are three times more likely than non-smokers to have prematurely aged skin, and even passive smokers may suffer. US research shows

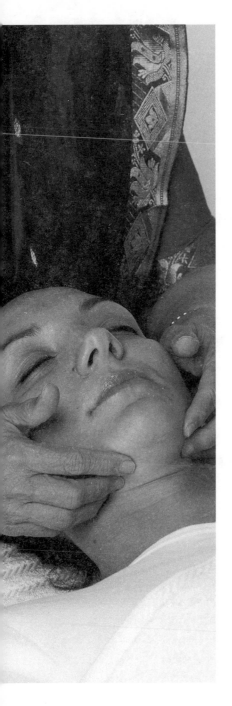

that smoking just 10 cigarettes a day for two years can double the number of wrinkles you get. A forty-year-old woman who has smoked for twenty years can look older than a sixty-year-old non-smoker. Cigarettes affect the skin in various ways. For example:

- ❁ *Cigarettes produce carbon monoxide, which occupies the red blood cells and limits the amount of oxygen that reaches the skin. Over the years the reduced oxygen supply makes the skin thinner, more lined, and leathery.*
- ❁ *Smoking destroys vitamin C, so delaying skin repair and renewal and increasing free-radical damage.*
- ❁ *The facial expressions associated with smoking, such as squinting and puckering the lips, tend to stretch delicate areas of the face.*
- ❁ *Inhaled smoke contains many noxious chemicals that damage collagen, elastin, and other connective tissue proteins. The skin thins by up to 40 percent, which allows water to escape more easily and encourages wrinkles. In addition, cadmium in cigarette smoke makes the skin dry and scaly.*

giving up

If giving up smoking permanently seems an impossible task, try it for a shorter time of, say, a month. You'll notice a big difference in the way you look and feel and this may be sufficient incentive to continue to give up.

If you really can't quit then at least try to cut down your intake, increase your consumption of water, and eat plenty of foods that are rich in vitamin C.

safety in the sun

Sunlight can be beneficial to the skin, as well as aiding general health and mental well-being. But overexposure is extremely damaging. Sunburn is a sign that serious tissue damage has occurred and can also lead to a greatly increased risk of skin cancer and premature skin aging. Damage caused by excessive sun exposure – known as photo-aging – can accumulate over the years, and takes a heavy toll.

There are two types of ultraviolet (UV) ray that can damage the skin. UVB rays make up about 20 percent of the solar radiation that reaches the Earth's surface, especially in the summer, and are the prime cause of sunburn and skin cancer. UVA rays account for the remaining 80 percent and can be a problem all year round, even in winter. They pass through the epidermis and deep into the dermis, damaging collagen and elastin fibers in the skin. UVA rays are also emitted by sunbeds but at much higher levels than that found in natural sunlight. So, while tanning machines are less likely to cause sunburn than sunbathing, they can cause greater damage to the supporting fibers, leading to premature wrinkling and sagging skin, in other words, speeding up the aging process. The best way to avoid this and keep skin looking younger for longer is to avoid sunbeds, limit the time spent in strong sunshine, and always use an appropriate sunscreen or sun-block.

sun protection

The pigment melanin in the skin helps to guard against sunburn, photo-aging, and skin cancer, so the lighter your skin, the greater the risk of sun damage. Fair-skinned people – especially blondes and red-heads – should take extra care. But even darker-skinned people need some protection against the aging effects of solar rays.

- ✿ *Avoid excessive exposure to the sun when the UV rays are strongest – between 11am and 3pm.*
- ✿ *Apply sunscreen 30 minutes before going outside to give it time to start working. In strong sunshine, apply every two hours. Use it liberally on the face and neck.*
- ✿ *In strong sunshine, wear a broad-brimmed hat to protect the face and neck.*
- ✿ *Wear sunglasses to prevent cataracts and to protect the delicate skin around the eyes, which is particularly prone to photo-aging.*
- ✿ *Eat plenty of fruit and vegetables rich in vitamin C as strong sunlight quickly depletes the skin's store of this protective chemical.*
- ✿ *Apply moisturizer liberally to the skin whenever you have been out in strong sunshine.*

which sun protection factor?

A sun protection factor (SPF) indicates how long you can safely stay in the sun without burning. For example, if your bare skin normally reddens after ten minutes in the sun then a sunscreen marked SPF8 protects your skin for up to 80 minutes (ie. 8 x 10). The general rule is the paler the skin, the quicker you'll burn and so the higher the SPF you'll need to stay safe. You should reapply sunscreen after swimming, or in very hot weather, when some protection is lost through sweating.

UV index

Many television stations and newspapers publish a daily solar UV index. This is a number between 1 and 20 that indicates the risk of sunburn. The index is based on the position of the sun in the sky and the level of cloud cover. During the summer months, especially, take notice of the solar UV index so you'll know when you are in greatest need of protection.

Skin types

Dermatologists have classified six skin types
to help you identify which SPF you need.

❀ Type 1: Naturally pale skin with a fine texture and a
translucent quality – typically red-heads and very fair-haired
"Nordic" types. It reddens within 10 minutes of exposure to
sunlight and quickly burns in strong sun. It never develops a
proper tan and peels after burning.

❀ Type 2: Naturally fair skin with a tendency to freckle –
typically, fair-haired blue-eyed people. When exposed to
strong sun it burns in about 20 minutes. Some tanning occurs
after repeated sun exposure.

❀ Type 3: Medium-toned skin, neither olive nor fair – typically,
dark-haired and brown-eyed people. This skin type tans fairly
easily and doesn't readily burn or freckle.

❀ Type 4: Olive tone, Mediterranean look – typically, very dark
brown- or black-haired people. This skin type tans easily and
doesn't often burn or freckle. But it still needs protection as
UV rays penetrate deep into skin.

✿ Type 5: Naturally brown skin – typically, people of Asian, North African or Middle Eastern origin. The skin almost never burns and darkens quickly on exposure to the sun. Nevertheless, some protection is recommended to guard against wrinkling.

✿ Type 6: Naturally dark-brown or black skin – typically, people of African origin. This skin type never burns and the skin darkens quickly on exposure to the sun. However, in very strong sunshine it will benefit from some sun protection to guard against wrinkling.

Sun protection factor chart

Type	1	2	3	4	5	6
UK/N. Europe	10–15	10–12	8–10	6–8	6	4–6
Mediterranean	15–20	12–15	10–12	8–10	6–8	6
Tropics/Africa	20–30	15–25	12–20	10–15	8–10	6–8

glossary

antioxidants: molecules that help protect against heart disease, cancer, and premature aging by neutralizing destructive atoms called free radicals.

aura: the sphere of spiritual energy that surrounds all living creatures. It is visible to mystics as a ball of white or colored light.

Ayurveda: an Indian system of preventative health care dating back 5000 years. The name is Sanskrit and literally means the "science of life."

Chakra: the term used to describe the body's energy centers. The literal meaning is "wheel" or "vortex." There are seven principal chakras.

collagen: the most abundant protein in the body, found in all connective tissue, including ligaments and tendons, and in bone. Much of the skin is made up of fibers of this material, for strength and flexibility.

dermis: underlying layer of the skin, containing connective tissue, blood vessels, glands, nerve fibers, and hair follicles.

dermatitis: inflammation of the skin, often in the form of a rash, red scales or flaking. It can be caused by a sensitivity to nickel, or chemicals such as soap, detergents, or skincare products, or by infection, stress or allergy.

doshas: the three complex elements or bioforces – called vata, pita, and kapha – that make up a person's constitution, or prakruti.

elastin: highly elastic protein material found in connective tissue, such as the dermis layer of the skin.

epidermis: top layer of skin, containing rapidly growing and dividing cells that flatten out and die as they approach the surface to form a protective barrier against damage and disease.

free radicals: highly destructive atoms that can damage living cells, causing heart disease, cancer, and premature aging. They are produced by cigarette smoking, sunbathing, frying foods, pollution, and as a by-product of normal chemical reactions in the cells.

ground substance: the non-fibrous protein that occupies the spaces between the collagen and elastin fibers of the skin's dermis layer. It is also known as the extracellular matrix.

keratin: hard-wearing protein that is the main component of hair, nails, and the epidermis layer of the skin.

lymph: straw-colored fluid that flows through a network of vessels called the lymphatic system. It transports fats around the body and also removes waste products from the tissues.

meridian: the channels through which the body's qi, or life force, flows. Stimulating the meridians, by means of acupressure for example, can relieve blockages and restore health.

polarity therapy: a healing system in which the therapist uses the power of touch to unblock points of stagnation in the body's energy flow and so restore balance.

prana: the Hindi word for universal life force or energy; equivalent to qi in Chinese Medicine.

protein: the main structural material in the body, forming the bulk of muscles and other tissues. It is also a vital constituent of the diet, needed for tissue growth, renewal, and repair.

qi: also known as chi, the universal life force that flows through the body along special pathways or channels. See meridians.

sebum: an oily substance produced by the sebaceous glands in the skin. It keeps the skin supple and lubricated and helps protect against moisture loss.

index

Make
www.thorsonselement.com
your online sanctuary

Get online information, inspiration and
guidance to help you on the path to physical
and spiritual well-being. Drawing on the integrity
and vision of our authors and titles, and with
health advice, articles, astrology, tarot, a
meditation zone, author interviews and events
listings, www.thorsonselement.com is a great
alternative to help create space and peace
in our lives.

So if you've always wondered about practising
yoga, following an allergy-free diet, using the
tarot or getting a life coach, we can point you
in the right direction.

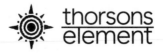

www.thorsonselement.com

3